IN AMERICA, we spend over 2.6 trillion dollars on health care each year, yet we rank 37th in the world for health care outcomes. Even more shocking, 50 million Americans don't have any sort of health insurance and another 80 million are underinsured. These harrowing statistics reflect that, as a nation, we focus more on disease and sickness than on wellness and health, creating a society where many are living sick and dying young.

The reality is clear: we suffer from a dysfunctional, have versus have-not health care system where medical miracles are performed for some, while access to care is denied to others. In Fractured, Dr. Epperly draws on his decades of experience as a family physician to identify the system's gaps and disparities and propose a compelling strategy to mend them, with the goal of creating an integrated, accessible, patient-centered approach to health and medicine.

The following questions will be tackled: What's wrong with the way we currently view, delivery, and pay for health care in America? What is our history of health care reform? How does our system compare to other nations? What can we do to fix health care now?

PRAISE FOR FRACTURED

"Dr. Epperly nails the diagnosis, bluntly calling out the travesty of pretending that the U.S. has a health care system when it actually has a wealth care system. His balanced analysis calls for all of us to recalibrate our thinking about how health is won and lost, and how the U.S. can regain a position of positive leadership in the world by crossing our arbitrary boundaries and working together to achieve stunning care and better health for all."

– Larry A. Green, MD, Professor and Epperson Zorn Chair for Innovation in Family Medicine and Primary Care, University of Colorado Denver

"In medicine a compound fracture is one in which the broken bone protrudes through the skin. This is an apt description of the U.S. health care system as described in *Fractured*. Dr. Epperly takes the wonder out of how to fix the problem. While not all of his steps are easy, with the people's commitment, they will create a clear path to the sustainable health care system we all seek."

– Don Kemper, MPH, Founder of Healthwise

"As a 'front line' physician with extensive experience in health care policy, Dr. Epperly outlines the primary causative factors for our dysfunctional system. This primer on what's wrong with health care and a path to a well-designed system is comprehensible to the layperson and those experienced in health care policy."

– Lori Heim, MD, Former President and Chairman of the Board, American Academy of Family Physicians

PRAISE FOR FRACTURED

"*Fractured* tells the gripping story of 'Richland' and 'Poorland'—a bifurcated United States where socioeconomic status determines life...and death. To call our current organization of U.S. health care a 'system' is an oxymoron that *Fractured* exposes. This book clearly highlights what's wrong with our U.S. health care system and provides a prescription for its reform."

– Jeff Susman, MD, Dean of the College of Medicine, Northeast Ohio Medical University and Editor of *Journal of Family Practice*

"In *Fractured*, Dr. Epperly uses stories and plain-speak to evidence the poor shape of the U.S. health care system accessible to the public. He fills an important gap, speaking to both policymakers and the public, explaining why the U.S. cannot afford to continue to do health care as it does now, not financially, not ethically."

– Robert L. Phillips, Jr., MD, MSPH, Director of the Robert Graham Center, Washington, D.C.

"*Fractured* provides a North Star for these leaders where their efforts will drive the sea change necessary to make America's entire health system be world class end to end."

– Dave Chase, CEO of Avado

"Dr. Ted Epperly brings a quarter century of expertise as a family physician and medical educator to his new book entitled *Fractured: America's Broken Health Care System and What We Must Do To Heal It*. The book is a clearly written and engaging description of the problems of America's health care system. Dr. Epperly has a knack of describing complex issues in easily understood stories. His book will be of use to anyone seeking to understand the reasons behind the current health care reform debate."

– John Saultz, MD, Professor and Chairman, Department of Family Medicine, Oregon Health and Science University

FRACTURED

*America's Broken Health Care System
and What We Must Do to Heal It*

by

Ted Epperly, MD

Paperback Edition
ISBN: 978-0-9916050-0-2

Cover design by Nick Lengua
Book design and edited by Greg Armstrong,
Michelle Robin, and Rachel Trusheim

10 9 8 7 6 5 4 3 2 1

Printed in the United States of America

Contents

Acknowledgments

To write a book of this scope and complexity takes many good people with skills beyond my own. The place to start in thanking those that have contributed to my book and made positive differences in its outcome is by thanking Greg Armstrong, PhD. Greg is a retired physicist who is the best technical editor I have ever worked with. His insight, wording suggestions, and ability to take three paragraphs and reduce it to two while keeping the content vibrant and enhancing the clarity is phenomenal. Whatever success I attain with this book I share with Greg for his time, energy, and expertise.

I cannot thank enough my wife, Lindy, who has been with me every step of the way through my development and growth as a physician but also my development and growth as an author. Her encouragement, feedback, editing, and late night and early morning discussions around the ideas in this book have been invaluable.

Thanks to my two sons, Morgan and Avery, who are never afraid to put their father in his place but also helped me with their encouragement and support. Morgan helped me develop by title. Avery helped me develop my webpage.

David Schmitz, MD; Jim Girvan, PhD, MPH; Mary McColl; Julie Robinson, DPA; Rick Kellerman, MD; Kara Cadwallader, MD; and Alan Rister all provided excellent edits and suggestions to early drafts of the book that were very helpful.

As can be imagined, there are many facts, details, and data on a topic as technical and complex as our health care system and its underlying strengths and weaknesses. I owe many thanks to the thoughts, knowledge, and expertise of Leslie Champlin, Kevin Burke, Kent Moore, Sarah Thomas, Cynthia Stapp, Janelle Davis, Rosi Sweeney, John Swanson, Teresa Baker, Jerome Connolly, Susan Hildebrandt, Hope Wittenberg, Laura Schmidt, Gail Jones, Denise Chuckovich, Russ Duke, Donna Valponi, Todd Dicus, Don Kemper, Dave Chase, and Drs Lori Heim, Roland Goertz, Glen Stream, Jeff Cain, Doug Henley, Robert Graham, Bob Phillips, Paul Grundy, Bob Crittenden, Perry Pugno, Norm Kahn, Dan Ostergaard, John Saultz, Frank Celestino, Pete Kozisek, Justin Glass, Amy McIntyre, Derek Jackson, Jim Blackman, Larry Green, Cal Gutkin, Rich Roberts, Chris van Weel, Jeff Susman, Fitz Mullen, and Scott Moser.

Finally, without the excellent technical assistance of Suzette Ansay, Michelle Robin, and Melanie Parish this book would have never been created. I cannot thank you enough for your commitment of effort and time in manuscript preparation and assistance in table and figure creation to turn this jumble of writing into a book of merit.

To the family physicians of our nation;
your excellent care of your patients
and your communities provides the foundation
on which tomorrow's health care
system will be built

and

To Lindy, Morgan, Avery, Mom,
and Greg, the rest of my family, and to the
residents, faculty and staff at the Family Medicine
Residency of Idaho who have made
all the work of this book worth it

It was the best of times, it was the worst of times,
it was the age of wisdom, it was the age of foolishness …

– Charles Dickens, *A Tale of Two Cities*

Chapter 1

THE FROG AND THE BOILING POT

We live in times of great change in the United States. These times provide crises but also great opportunity. Health care is close to the beating heart of every American. Our efforts over the last several years to correct major flaws in our health care system have transcended policy reform only to be mired down with the spin of politics, media, blogs, and talk-show hosts. There has been much confusion, anger, myths, lies, and fear around reforming our badly fractured and broken health care system. I have come to learn that a confused mind takes refuge in the word no. An informed and educated mind, on the other hand, will thoughtfully evaluate the possibilities, alternatives, and opportunities. My goal in writing this book is to educate as many people as possible on the current state of our nation's health care system: why it is fractured and what we must do to heal it. We have together created what may be the best nation in the history of the world. Our Founding Fathers brought into existence a wonderful country, one built on freedom. It was their collective vision—along with our inherited drive to pursue life, liberty, and justice for all—that has made our young nation greater than the sum of its parts. It gave us a country to be proud of and a nation that has made many positive changes in the world. The United States has led the way with tremendous innovation and creativity to help transform the world from the Agricultural Age to the Industrial Age, and now to the Information Age. In many ways we have answered the call for progress.

Despite these advancements in science and technology, our nation's health care system has faltered. Though we spend $2.6 trillion on health care each year in America, two to four times higher per person than the health care costs in any other industrialized nation, we rank 37th in the world for our health care outcomes, such as life expectancy, infant mortality, or immunization rates. We rank 54th in the world for having a fair, just, and equitable health care system. Not only is it wildly expensive, but we also have major gaps in quality and glaring disparities of care for our citizens. Fifty million people living in the United States don't have any sort of health insurance and another 80 million are underinsured (1). We have settled for a "have" and "have-not" health care system, where the "have-nots" live sick and die young.

Why then has it been such a struggle to seek a better health care system? Why haven't we ensured that health care for all is a basic right? Why have we hesitated to reach out with an open hand to guarantee that basic health care is accessible to all in need? Why would we as a country not want all of our people to have the best opportunity to lead healthy lives?

This book was written to analyze these questions and provide insight and answers to this perplexing paradox. On one hand, we have valued our important ethic of being our brother's keeper by embracing the concept of caring for all. On the other hand, we have a fiercely independent, competitive spirit that takes no prisoners and revels in the mantra of pulling ourselves up by our own bootstraps. Where do we find the balance between these two ideologies?

The poet Maya Angelou said, "There is no greater agony than bearing an untold story inside of you." Therefore, allow me to tell you a bit about my personal story of how I became interested in health care reform and health care policy. My involvement began because of a transition I made from the United States Army into the general public's medical health care system. For 21 years I was an Army family physician. I worked and acted as part of a team that focused on high-quality, patient-centered health care. There was not much difference in compensation among the categories of physicians we had in the military, and we were all on a salaried payment system.

The dynamic was established around serving our patients, with no further income being generated by the system for us as individuals. Everyone was seen in a timely manner and received great medical care, be they private or general. Disparities in care were minimized and quality of care maximized. When I transitioned into the civilian health care system in July of 2001, I was plunged into an environment where that dynamic did not exist. The system was greedy, driven by revenue generation, and divided by the haves and have-nots. I was deeply troubled.

You may have heard of the story of the frog in the pot of water. As the story goes, if a frog is kept in a pot of water and the temperature is slowly raised to boiling, the frog will not jump out of the pot and will boil to death. However, if a frog is thrown into an already boiling pot of water, it will immediately jump out. I suddenly realized that I was that frog. I had worked in a system for 21 years where health care was provided to all and service to others was our orientation; in a system where we did not profit because of someone's misfortune; where resources were applied to keep people healthy, not just to treat them when they became sick or injured. I had then been thrown into a boiling pot: an unfamiliar system of health care that was a business not a profession and where not everyone was afforded basic care; where access to health care was not a given; where wide disparities in health care were obvious; a system in which people just assumed that this is the way health care is delivered. I had just left the "military-industrial complex," where the federal government, the United States military, and defense contractors have created a multibillion-dollar industry. Yet this was an even larger and more expensive industry: the "medical-industrial complex." Instead of being priced at hundreds of billions of dollars per year, this health care industry was an unfathomable $2.6 trillion per year.

I was shocked by the monumental differences between these two health care systems. It was a hard slap across my face; my first wake-up call. The stark contrast between these two systems of care made me decide to take the bold step forward of trying to determine what issues were at the root of the problem. What could possibly and re-alistically be done to help our nation transform a tremendously com-plex, expensive health care system (one that is bankrupting individu-als, families, businesses, states, and our country) into one that better serves the health care of our people and our nation? I decided to join a movement to change our health care system from what we *have* to what America *needs*. I naively assumed that everyone would certainly want these changes as well. Why wouldn't they? Why wouldn't we all want a health care system that provides timely access to affordable, high-quality health care; one that would help us all live healthier, more productive lives? After all, this is how a physician typically thinks. This is when my second wake-up call occurred.

I attended a town hall meeting on health care reform hosted by the citizens of my hometown in Boise, Idaho, in August of 2009. At that time, the health care debate was starting to get ugly, personal, political, and mean-spirited all across America, and the Tea Party Coalition had come out in force to this particular town hall meet-ing. I was shocked by not only this health care reform meeting but at countless others that were occurring all across our nation. I was amazed that something as basic as evolving our fractured, expensive, bloated, and poorly performing health care system would be subject to so much anger, lies, hate, and fear. I was dumbfounded at the distor-tions of truth and at the basic misunderstandings underlying much of what was being proposed within both the Senate and House health care reform bills. Since I had spent the last seven years closely work-ing on these issues, it was disappointing to see that people saw this as a government takeover of health care; that they doggedly maintained the belief that the resulting cost of reform was too expensive and so let's just leave health care alone and maintain the status quo. It was the name-calling, the hissing from the crowd, the fists being shaken in anger, the outright threats of harm to people, and the expression of palpable fear that made me decide to write this book. My purpose is to educate and to better explain what is going on with our health care system. My goal is not to take one political side or another, nor judge who is right or wrong. We need to clarify what is fractured in our massive health care system and help people better understand what our collective responsibilities are in trying to heal it.

Carved into the wall of the Health and Human Services building in Washington, D.C., where the headquarters of our nation's Medicare and Medicaid programs stands, is this quote by Hubert H. Humphrey from November 1, 1977: "The moral test of a government is how that government treats those in the dawn of life—the children; the twilight of life—the elderly; and the shadows of life—the sick, the needy, and the handicapped." Health care for all is a mirror for who we are as a people, a culture, and a nation. *Fractured: America's Broken Health Care System and What We Must Do To Heal It* analyzes what is fundamentally flawed about our health care system and identifies a path that will lead us to a much better future. Indeed, our nation's present journey to change our fractured health care system provides a penetrating look into the very essence of America. In order to fix it, we must first come to a clear diagnosis about what our problems are. The next chapter will examine what is wrong with our health care system.

Chapter 2

WHAT IS WRONG WITH OUR HEALTH CARE SYSTEM?

All of us enjoy the many benefits of living in our great nation. Freedom, choice, security, and opportunity are but a few of the advantages we share as Americans. Many of us claim that among these benefits we have the best health care system in the world. However, this is sadly not the case. We have gaps in health care quality across our population, leading to a widely divergent "have" and "have-not" health care system; one that produces only mediocre health outcomes when compared to the rest of the world (1, 2). Why does the United States of America continue to trudge along with an inefficient, costly, complex, and hard-to-access system when many other industrialized countries do not? What is it about our uniquely American health care system that is fractured?

Now, to be balanced and fair, there are many things right with our health care system. We have tremendous depth and specialization in all areas of medicine. Our research—generating new knowledge, technology, and innovation—is breathtaking. Our spending on health care is unrivaled anywhere else on the planet. Our magnificent hospitals are gleaming megaliths of steel and glass, fortified by an armada of specialists. These institutions house polished operating rooms, surgical robots, and the latest and greatest MRI and PET scanners.

Thus, we have a puzzle. Why does our nation fumble when trying to translate a tour de force of knowledge, technology, money, and skill into high-quality health care? To underline existing problems with our health care system, I will explore three major questions: What's wrong with our current view of health care? What's wrong with the way we pay for health care? What's wrong with the way we deliver health care?

Let's examine what is wrong with our current view of health care.

LACK OF FOCUS ON HEALTH

Perhaps the most important answer is that we are captivated by the wrong end of health care. We are absorbed with disease rather than health. The American health care system is more known for doing things to people after disease occurs than it is for preventing such needs by taking action beforehand. If we were truly focused on health instead of disease, we would reward behaviors that promote health (exercise, nutrition, smoking cessation, etc.), rather than merely treating disease reflexively (procedures, imaging, and high-end technology).

Why are we so focused on disease? There are five main reasons:

1. Our health care system doesn't pay health care professionals to nurture health. It pays them to treat disease, illness, and injury. To understand our health care system, all we need to do is follow the flow of money. The money is in disease, not in promoting health.

2. Our medical schools and health care teaching institutions concentrate on diseases, their pathologies, and the wondrous science of medicine that treats them. Our training model is biased strongly toward disease and minimally toward its prevention. We spend hardly any time in medical and nursing school on the importance of exercise, nutrition, diet, sleep, stress reduction, emotional health, smoking cessation, alcohol moderation, and other determinants of health.

3. Talking about health isn't nearly as much fun, or as exciting, as talking about stamping out disease or saving a life.

It's much more interesting to talk about the snap diagnosis of bacterial endocarditis, the fascinating aortic aneurysm surgery, or doing a colonoscopy and finding cancer in the sigmoid colon. It is not as dramatic to talk about a diet and exercise plan to lose 25 pounds, even though this is an excellent tactic to prevent or delay the development of hypertension, diabetes, or degenerative arthritis of the knees and hips.

4. It is simply easier to do something to someone than to prevent the problem from happening in the first place. Doctors like to do things. As a doctor, I want to feel needed, be useful, and make a difference in a patient's life. When your only tool is a hammer, then everything looks like a nail. Using this metaphor, there are a lot of "nails" sticking up across the country waiting for our doctors to hammer down and we are well paid to do so. In contrast, it is a complex task to induce people with entrenched and damaging personal habits to change their behaviors for the sake of their health. And worse yet, our health care system pays doctors hardly anything to focus aggressively on these issues. The skill needed to educate and inspire compliance to good health habits only comes through time and the development of a trusting relationship with the patients you are treating. If you don't have the time or the ability or the relationship, then this is poorly done, or not done at all.

5. By doing something for people there is a sense of instant gratification. A surgery, a diagnosis, a test, an x-ray, a prescription, or a procedure are all events that can be easily observed. Dealing with health and prevention is a delayed gratification often spanning years or decades, and only appreciated over time.

The analysis of healthcare provides a continuum that can be observed:

Figure 1. Continuum of Health to Disease and its Associated Cost

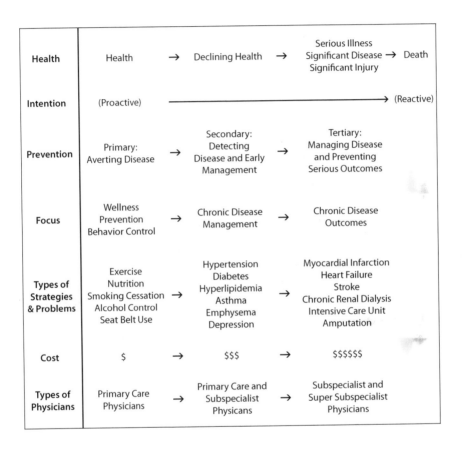

Health	Health → Declining Health →		Serious Illness Significant Disease → Death Significant Injury
Intention	(Proactive) ────────────────────────→ (Reactive)		
Prevention	Primary: Averting Disease →	Secondary: Detecting Disease and Early Management →	Tertiary: Managing Disease and Preventing Serious Outcomes
Focus	Wellness Prevention Behavior Control →	Chronic Disease Management →	Chronic Disease Outcomes
Types of Strategies & Problems	Exercise Nutrition Smoking Cessation → Alcohol Control Seat Belt Use	Hypertension Diabetes Hyperlipidemia → Asthma Emphysema Depression	Myocardial Infarction Heart Failure Stroke Chronic Renal Dialysis Intensive Care Unit Amputation
Cost	$ →	$$$ →	$$$$$$
Types of Physicians	Primary Care Physicians →	Primary Care and Subspecialist → Physicans	Subspecialist and Super Subspecialist Physicians

On the far left of the line is the front end of health, where prevention, wellness, and primary care reside. As we go from left to right across the line, we get to the back end of health care, where disease and injury exist, and where things are done to people in our reactive sick care system. We will reluctantly pay pennies on the dollar on the front end of health care to encourage wellness, prevention, and health promotion, and yet we will pay tens to hundreds of thousands of dollars on the back end of health care to provide heart attack treatment, stroke treatment, chronic renal dialysis, neonatal intensive care for premature babies, and limb amputations resulting from uncontrolled diabetes. We have lost our willingness to set rational priorities about what we should do for the people of this country. Our goal should be to keep them healthy and thus avoid procedures, rather than to settle for a system that only treats people when maladies have occurred.

We have created a medical-industrial complex (fueled by $2.6 trillion per year) to do things to people, blocking attention from the type of health care that would have prevented those things from being necessary in the first place. What health problems do the majority of people die from in the United States? The vast majority of causes are related to the individuals' health behaviors. Indeed, 40 percent of these deaths are tied to obesity, diet, nutrition, lack of exercise, smoking, excessive alcohol drinking, lack of seat belts, and the like (3, 4). Thirty percent of deaths are related to one's genetics, 15 percent to socioeconomic conditions, 10 percent to a medical-care-related issue, and 5 percent to one's environment. Only 5 percent to 8 percent of these items are impacted by our nation's health care expenditures each year. The rest of our health care spending (92 percent to 95 percent) goes to items that have a relatively minor effect on the health determinants of people or the overall health of our nation (3, 4). These monies pay for surgeries, procedures, imaging, medications, medical devices, hospitalizations, emergency room care, and intensive care. These items are extremely important for the individual but actually should not be at the top of the health care priority list for the nation as a whole.

Figure 2 displays what happens in our nation during an average month in terms of health care.

Figure 2. What Happens to Patients in an Average Month

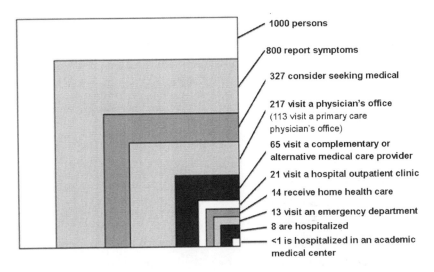

1000 persons

800 report symptoms

327 consider seeking medical

217 visit a physician's office
(113 visit a primary care
physician's office)

65 visit a complementary or
alternative medical care provider

21 visit a hospital outpatient clinic

14 receive home health care

13 visit an emergency department

8 are hospitalized

<1 is hospitalized in an academic
medical center

Sources:

White KL, Williams TF, Greenberg BG. The ecology of medical care. N Engl J Med 1961;265:885-892.

Green LA, Fryer GE, Yawn BP, Lanier D, Dovey SM. The ecology of medical care revisited. N Engl J Med 2001;344:2021-2025.

As can be seen in this diagram, for every 1,000 people, 800 (80 percent) will report some sort of health-related symptoms and 327 (32.7 percent) will consider seeking some sort of medical care in an average month. Two hundred and seventeen (21.7 percent) will visit a physician's office, with only about half of those 113 (11.3 percent) seeing a primary care physician. Sixty-five (6.5 percent) will see a complimentary or alternative medical care provider (e.g., a chiropractor, naturopath, etc.), and 21 (2.1 percent) will visit a hospital-based ambulatory clinic. Fourteen (1.4 percent) will receive home health care. Thirteen (1.3 percent) will visit an emergency room, 8 will be hospitalized (0.8 percent), and less than one (0.1 percent) will end up in an academic medical center. The frightening reality is that the small number of people (2.1 percent) who visit emergency rooms or are admitted as inpatients at hospitals and large academic medical centers account for 92 percent of all the money spent on health care each year in the United States. That statistic is staggering.

This data was first observed in 1961 by White et al. (5), and reconfirmed 40 years later by Green et al. (6). With this in mind, *where* is the majority of money spent on health care? *Where* are the majority of physicians located? *Where* are the majority of physicians trained? The answer may surprise you. They are trained in the academic teaching hospitals of medical schools. They are trained in the operating rooms, the intensive care units, the neonatal intensive care units, the hospital medical and surgical wards, and in hospital emergency rooms. They are not trained in the community offices of physicians, health departments, or community health centers.

Our nation focuses on the back end of health care; on the high-dollar, high-cost areas loaded with technology. These areas are sexy and spawn TV shows like *Grey's Anatomy* and *House*. They also breed the deluge of TV ads that steer you towards the latest and greatest pharmaceutical medications. The ads make it sound as if you must have this medication to live a happy, satisfied, and productive life, even though you may never need these medications, and for which there are most likely cheaper, equally effective medications on the market. But what about all the other areas in the figure? This is the province of prevention, health promotion, wellness, chronic disease management, primary care, and good outpatient, community-based ambulatory care. This is the arena of promoting health and wellness and keeping people away from the hospitals. This is what tomorrow's health care system must focus on. We must focus on *health* and not *disease*.

We must also focus on leveraging resources in the community and in families to promote health, and only utilize emergency rooms and hospitals and the high-cost palaces of our health care system when the above strategies fail or an accident happens. In fact, most of the important decisions regarding health care in our nation are not made by physicians, nurses, or health insurance companies at all. They are made by the women of America: mothers, wives, and—in families caring for an aged family member—daughters. These decisions occur in communities and in homes all across America. Our health care system and our primary care providers must engage these women in proactive ways to assist in good health decisions. Can you only imagine the impact on the health of our nation if we were to proactively support the good decisions women make on behalf of their families and give them the tools to make even better choices?

To recap, it is a lack of focus on health, and simultaneously an intense focus on disease and its treatment that have driven major shortcomings in America's health care system. What America is known for is having, perhaps, the best-reactive, most-expensive "sick care" system in the world!

LACK OF PATIENT-CENTEREDNESS

Much of America's health care system is not built on what is good for people: accessibility, timely care, quality care, service-oriented care, and having a personal physician who knows your ongoing health care challenges. This is not to imply that the providers and members of our health care teams are not good people; they are indeed outstanding people. The problem is that the patient is not at the center of our system. What *is* at the center of our system are the physicians, hospitals, pharmaceutical companies, and medical industry delivering the care, and the health insurance companies paying for it. This creates a mind-set of medicine as a business, a wealth-generating system, instead of medicine as a profession and a health-generating system. It creates confusion and complexity instead of clarity and simplicity.

LACK OF COVERAGE

Part of the problem with the American health care system is that not everybody has affordable insurance or some type of health care coverage. There are over 50 million uninsured patients according to the United States Census Bureau (7). Of that 50 million, about 10 million are estimated to be illegal immigrants, 10 million are people who could afford insurance if they truly wanted it, and the remaining 30 million are people who want health care insurance but cannot afford it. In addition, there are approximately another 80 million Americans who are underinsured. This means they have limitations in their coverage or not enough health insurance to cover significant portions of their medical bills. This leads to our have and have-not health care system that is in part responsible for our poor health care outcomes. The Commonwealth Fund has shown that the two items that most consistently improve people's health care outcomes are health care insurance and a usual source of care (8). We must do a better job as a nation to get all of our people covered so that we can better direct them to the front end of our health care system, which targets wellness, health, behavioral changes, and shared health care responsibility. This contrasts to having a lack of access to health care, where people are constrained to utilize the system only when they're sicker and entering the higher-cost back end of health care by way of the emergency room, hospitalizations, and procedural care.

In addition, the expenses of the uninsured are being charged to them at full cost. This is in contrast to insured people, who have obtained their policies with rates negotiated by employers or insurance agents. These rates are lower than what hospitals or physicians may charge the uninsured. The uninsured get the full bill, not the negotiated lower cost bill that the insurance company has negotiated to pay. This bill can be 5 to 25 percent higher. If uninsured patients can't pay these bills, then this cost is shifted towards insurance companies, employers, and individual citizens. These costs appear as escalating premiums and costs that physicians, hospitals, health insurance companies, and health care systems charge to make up for the uncovered expenses of charity and bad debt. This is why it is imperative to get as many people in this country covered for health care as we possibly can. "Everyone in and nobody out" provides the greatest way to ensure an equitable distribution of benefits and costs to the population as a whole. To do this, America must be able to answer a fundamental question. Is health care a basic right or is it not? Is health care something all Americans should receive, or is it a money-based privilege? The answer to this question becomes essential in building our future health care system because it reveals our nation's values. We will talk more about this issue later in the book.

WHAT'S WRONG WITH THE WAY WE PAY FOR HEALTH CARE?

Cost

As previously mentioned, the cost of health care in our nation is $2.6 trillion per year. This represents 17 percent of our gross domestic product and is the largest single sector of the entire American economy (9). This cost is rapidly spiraling out of control. Figures 3 and 4 below reveal the rapid escalation of health care expenditures in this country.

Figure 3. National Health Spending in Billions

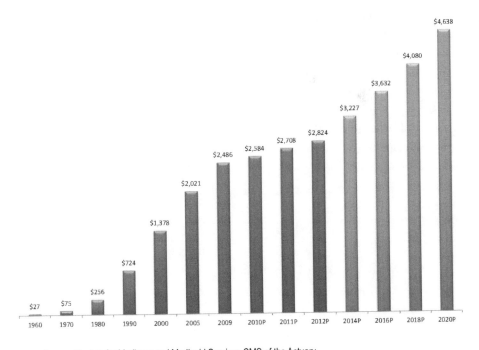

Source: Centers for Medicare and Medicaid Services CMS of the Actuary

Figure 4. Escalation of Gross Domestic Product Spending on Healthcare

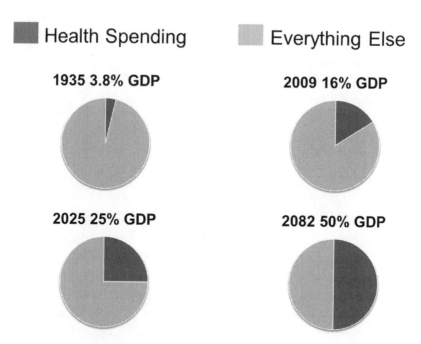

Source: Centers for Medicare & Medicaid Services. NHE Fact Sheet. [http://www.cms.hhs.gov/NationalHealthExpendData/25_NHE_Fact_Sheet.asp#TopOfPage]

If unchecked, the amount spent on health care dollars as a portion of the gross domestic product will go from 17 percent in 2009 to 25 percent in the year 2025, and 50 percent in the year 2082 (10). This cost escalation is a major threat. It is the specter that haunts the American health care system.

As our nation staggers under the financial cost of our health care system, it is also impacting individuals and their families. The number one reason for personal bankruptcy in our country is medical expense (11). Sixty-two percent of all United States bankruptcies in 2007 were related to medical expenses (12). The percentage of bankruptcies caused by medical problems rose by 50 percent between 2001 and 2007. The cost of health care is causing a personal bankruptcy every

30 seconds in America (13). And, when you analyze such bankrupt-cies, over 78 percent were filed by people who actually had medical insurance (12). This is particularly sad for America since other in-dustrialized countries do not have personal bankruptcies for medical bills. Not one of them. That is not how their systems are designed.

Similarly, when we analyze how this plays out on our nation's largest payer, Medicare, this program will become financially in-solvent in the year 2024 at its current rate of spending (14). This is particularly tragic because we now have 40 million Americans over the age of 65, and this will grow to be 80 million Americans over the age of 65 in the next 15 years (15). We must get cost under control or it will implode our economy. It is like swimming across a lake with a 40-pound rock tied to your body. You may be able to get 15 to 30 feet out from the shoreline, but you're not going to make it across the lake. You will ultimately be dragged down. President Obama said at his White House Summit on March 5, 2009, "One of the greatest threats, not just to the well-being of our families and the prosperity of our businesses but to the very foundation of our economy, is the exploding cost of health care in America today" (16). That's why bold steps must be taken now to right this ship and to bend the cost curve.

Payment Systems

America's health care system is steered by how physicians, hospitals, and other health care professionals get paid. Physicians get paid to do things to people. Physicians do not get paid to prevent illness or injury from happening to people. The incentives are all wrong. This has led to a system that values volume of care over good outcomes of care; quantity over quality. The fee-for-service system in American health care rewards physicians to test, to do procedures, to do imag-ing, and to overdo. The fee-for-service system is based on charging for your service each time you see a patient face-to-face. You see more people, you bill more. It has nothing to do with the accuracy or quality of what you do. The fee-for-service model only values that you see them. Therefore, the number of patients seen is what drives payment, not the outcomes or accuracy of what is produced by the encounter. Seeing a patient with hypertension or diabetes is what you get paid for. It is not whether you actually helped the patient or not. A primary care physician is similar to a hamster running on a wheel. Because primary care physician fees are lower than those of the subspecialists or proceduralists, and since seeing paying patients is what drives revenue, primary care physicians must run faster and faster to generate enough patient volume to drive enough payment to have enough margin to keep their practices alive and open. You may have noticed that in this scenario nobody is asking the question about the health care outcomes of the patients. Are they improving? Are they satisfied with the care they're getting? Is it making a difference? On the contrary, our health care system has been perfectly designed to give what a capitalistic health care system is meant to give. It is a system that provides what it gets paid to provide. It gets back to the question: where are the dollars invested in our health care system? The current answer is that they are invested on the back end of health care, not on the front end in terms of wellness, health care promotion, and prevention. If those front-end services paid more than those on the back end of health care, then we would see our system migrate to doing those things. It's a matter of priority; it's a matter of incentives; it's a matter of what we want from our health care system.

Another way in which the payment system has a major influence on the physician workforce is in the generation of differential incomes between types of physicians. Because our system preferentially pays subspecialists more to do procedures and imaging, it has undervalued and underpaid primary care physicians on the front end of health care—the very physicians who are trying to prevent back-end services from being necessary in the first place. As a result, we have created incomes that range between two and five times higher (or even more) for subspecialists than for primary care physicians (16). This leads to a tremendous fork in the road for medical students when deciding what types of physicians to become. The average medical student is now coming out of medical school with approximately $142,000 in medical school loans (17). When they then stand on the precipice of making a choice of whether or not to become a subspecialist, they see the salary differential between the different types of physicians, and they are strongly drawn to the subspecialties. This financial incentive has become a major factor in our health care system's make-up, and has resulted in a marked imbalance in the medical workforce in our country.

When we step outside of the United States and look at other industrialized countries, we see these nations' workforces at an approximate 50/50 balance in terms of subspecialists to primary care physicians. At the time of this writing, that ratio in the United States is 70 percent subspecialists to 30 percent generalists. If we look at what the nation's medical schools have produced over the last 10 years of training, approximately 90 percent of medical students are going into the subspecialties and only 10 percent into the primary care areas of family medicine, general internal medicine, or general pediatrics. This will have a major negative impact on the United States' ability to deliver comprehensive, integrated, coordinated, and accessible primary care at the front end of the health care system.

Health Insurance System

Our country's system of health insurance is not focused on health care. Our insurance system is focused on profitability to stockholders and minimizing financial risk. It is a paradox that employers and employees pay quite a bit for health care coverage, and then struggle to get the insurance system to pay for needed health care services. The insurance industry is much more absorbed with denying coverage, avoiding those with preexisting conditions, and limiting payment amounts to the very individuals they claim they serve. Basically, health insurance is costing more and covering less. It boils down to the average family not being able to afford the average premium. The average family makes about $48,000 in the United States and the average premium is $15,000 per year. This is up 9 percent from last year and is costing the average annual worker over $600 in increased premiums over the last two years (18). Family insurance is now costing each year more than a small car (19). According to the Kaiser Family Foundation, health insurance premiums have gone up by 113 percent while wages have increased by only 34 percent over the last 10 years (18). To add insult to injury, not only is health care insurance costing more, but at the same time it is less comprehensive, resulting in greater out-of-pocket spending. In fact, employers are having to choose between providing good benefits or higher pay for their employees and hiring new employees entirely. It is a problem when the profit margins of insurance companies are stuffed back into the pockets of stockholders, as opposed to being plowed back into the health care of their customers. I will talk more about the insurance industry later in the book.

Liability System

Although America has 5 percent of the world's population, it has 50 percent of the world's lawyers. In fact, there are 27 percent more lawyers in the United States than physicians (approximately 730,800 physicians in active practice compared to 1,143,000 lawyers). This produces a ratio of one physician for every 406 Americans but provides one lawyer for every 265 Americans (20). Our tort system reflects a very litigious-minded nation and this strongly affects health care. If physicians do not have a trusting relationship with their patients, they tend to practice defensive medicine and often over-order, over-diagnose, over-treat, and over-consult on patient care, driving up health care cost. Indeed, the estimate of the cost of defensive medicine is approximately $124 billion per year (21, 22). This is why primary care, in which there is a trusted, personal relationship, is so important. For subspecialists such a relationship usually does not exist. They are often seeing patients for the first time, interacting with them in the ER, meeting them in a hospital room, or seeing them as a referral in their office. This encourages a tendency to overdo, which is further incentivized by the fee-per-service system. When overdoing then aligns with ensuring that they don't get sued, it becomes a natural default condition for physicians in our health care system. More leads to more and costs continue to escalate. Having a trusting relationship with the patient by the physician can make saying "no, this is not needed" easier to do. The breakdown of personal relationships between physicians and patients has driven a large amount of business for America's trial lawyers. Malpractice cases have become an important line of work and a revenue generator for lawyers, and are part of what drives up the cost of health care.

WHAT'S WRONG WITH THE WAY WE DELIVER HEALTH CARE?

Lack of a Health Care System

Our nation's devotion to the back end of health care (as opposed to a front-end-oriented approach to wellness and health care) is compounded by not having an integrated and coordinated health care system. Our health care system in the United States is terribly fragmented. Hospitals, clinics, emergency rooms, physicians' offices, physicians, and health care systems do not integrate and share information well with each other. In fact, the system as a whole does not communicate effectively with different subsets of the system. It seems that we all work in our own vertical silos with minimal bridging of information from one physician to another or from one facility to another. I am constantly struck by the fact that I can use my ATM card to get cash from any bank's machine around the world within seconds, but I cannot communicate effectively with a clinic a block away about the care of my patient. Information about the patient should flow seamlessly across multiple settings in a secure manner that presents the health care provider with accurate, relevant, up-to-date knowledge and information, helping the patient and physician make effective choices and decisions about the patient's care.

Now don't get me wrong, we have incredibly talented and gifted physicians and health care teams in this country. In fact, I would say we have the best physicians anywhere in the world. But we don't work well together. It's like having the five best basketball players on the planet. According to our system of payment, we give each of them a basketball and tell them to dribble around and shoot at will. We tell them that every time they shoot the ball they will be paid. They don't even have to make the basket to get paid; they just need to shoot the ball. And so we have these five superstar basketball players dribbling and shooting constantly in a fragmented, nonintegrated, non-coordinated fashion. And to make matters worse, they don't communicate with each other in any effective way to modify their behavior for each other's aid, let alone their patient's. We then play a team from Spain, England, Canada, France, or Germany, and we get beat. Why? Not because we don't have the best basketball players on this planet; it is because we do not pass the ball and play as a team. When you step back and look at how our nation performs health care, we stack up poorly against the other industrialized nations in terms of outcomes. Not because we don't have talented people, but because we care for our patients using a fragmented, nonintegrated, unaccountable, nonfunctioning system of record-keeping and communication. It is not connected well with information sharing. Insurers and payers are locked into payment incentives that do not value teamwork. Our system does not presently pay you to work as a larger, integrated, and accountable team.

Part of our lack of integration and coordination is the failure to adopt electronic medical records en mass and a concurrent failure to leverage information technology systems. Although in almost all sectors of this country we are rapidly transforming our culture from the Industrial Age into the Information Age, medicine lags behind and struggles. In fact, I would submit that in terms of electronic medical records and information technology systems, medicine is still mired in the Industrial Age. We continue to fail to employ knowledge sharing at the point of service for patient care.

Lack of Primary Care

If we are going to cover as many people as possible, as was noted previously, we must have a health care system in the country that delivers integrated, coordinated primary care and is focused on wellness, chronic disease management, and prevention. If we don't have a robust primary care system that can deliver this care to all, then we effectively have no health care system. It would be like giving all the citizens of this nation free bus passes but only having two busses to put them on. It would be like giving all citizens free vouchers to go to restaurants to eat but only having two restaurants that they can utilize. In a system that is extremely skewed towards subspecialists, we are shorting America on the primary care workforce that it must have to deliver care (23). This is leading to a tremendous dilemma for our health care policy experts, Congress, and the nation as a whole. At a time when we are trying to expand coverage to all, we don't have the correct workforce mix among our physicians to provide that care. We don't have the right players on the court.

Why is the type of care provided by primary care physicians important? Primary care physicians are experts at providing acute, chronic, and preventative medical care in a timely way that keeps problems from getting worse or avoids the problems altogether. By having broad, comprehensive knowledge of the human body and of the person living in that body and his or her family, the physician knows how to deliver the right type of care tailored to that individual at the right time (see Figure 1). Primary care physicians provide people a trusting, personal relationship that educates and motivates them to follow their medical roadmap and to change their behaviors for long-term better health (recall that 40 percent of all deaths in our country relate to people's behavior). Such a partnership only happens over time through a continuing, shared relationship. It is the primary care physician that integrates and coordinates work from other physicians, the emergency room, hospitalizations, and other parts of the health care system into a plan of management for the patient. Primary care physicians connect the dots and provide patients a stable platform of care.

Evidence that health care systems function maximally when based on primary care is very well documented. The work of Barbara Starfield, the Commonwealth Fund, the Kaiser Family Foundation, the World Health Organization, Medicare data, and the Dartmouth Atlas' work of Medicare Health Care Costs have made it clear that as the number of primary care physicians go up in a community, health care costs come down and quality indicators go up (24, 25, 26). Morbidity and mortality are reduced and patient satisfaction increases. Indeed, there is a linear relationship between increasing primary care physician ratios and improving results on health care costs and outcomes (26). Conversely, as subspecialists go up in an area, health care costs increase and quality decreases. This is not because subspecialists are poor physicians. They are extremely good physicians, but they have a very narrow, limited, comprehensive skill set. When subspecialists get out of their areas of expertise, they tend to over-order tests, over-diagnose problems, over-image, and over-consult to other subspecialist colleagues. All of this has an additive effect, increasing health care costs and having more things done to the patient. This occurs due to their uncertainty over what to do in medical areas outside of their expertise, as well as to the fact that without a close, personal relationship with the patient they don't want to be sued for making a mistake. As Dr. Atul Gawande outlined in his article "Cost Conundrum" in the June issue 2009 of the *New Yorker* magazine, more health care is not always better health care (27). In fact, more health care can lead to bad outcomes and clearly more expensive costs. More leads to more! Supply drives demand. That is why every patient should have a primary care physician as their personal, trusted, health care physician. This provides an advocate for the patient and someone who has a global knowledge of the health care system, helping the patient understand what they need and, more importantly, what they do not need.

Poor Health Outcomes

Despite the fact that we spend more on health care than any other nation in the world at approximately $8,500 per year for every man, woman, and child in this country, our health care outcomes do not stack up as the best in the world. We have a strong disconnect between what we spend for health care and what we get back in health care outcomes. Despite the fact that we spend $2.6 trillion per year on health care, far more than any other country in the world, we rank 37th in the world for health care outcomes and 54th in the world for a fair, just, and equitable system (25). In a recent study done by the Commonwealth Fund, the United States ranked 19th out of 19 countries in regards to mortality amenable to medical care (2).

This failure in outcomes stems from the factors that I have repeated throughout this chapter. We must integrate and coordinate our health care system. We must cover our people and have a primary care-based system on which to build our health care system. By having trusting relationships with physicians who can coordinate health care and focus on the front end of health care (prevention, wellness, and health care promotion), we can start to bend the cost curve and improve health care outcomes for the good of the nation.

Medical Schools

The nation's 135 medical schools that produce MD (doctors of medicine) physicians and 26 osteopathic schools that produce DOs (doctors of osteopathy) select, through rigorous admissions policies, students who are bright and capable. Medical students are trained in the first two years of medical or osteopathic school in a very reductionistic training model. They are trained to drill down on a "micromodel" level to data emerging from cellular physiology, embryology, anatomy, histology, biochemistry, and pathology. These students are trained in a disease model. Medical school admissions committees in the United States select students who tend to align with reductionistic thinking. The problem is that much of what health care is about is not centered on reductionistic thinking but rather holistic thinking based on service to people. Medical care is about treating a whole person in the context of their family and their community. It is not about treating disease. It is about treating a person with a disease. That bigger ("macro") view at the globalized holistic scale is not done well in medical schools with their "micro" view education model. Therefore, the products of much of medical school training are reductionistic thinkers who align very well with becoming subspecialists: partialists instead of generalists. They are not usually holistic thinkers who align well with comprehensive service to a person, their family, and their community. Again, if your focus is only on a particular organ, gender, or disease process, you tend to limit physicians who are more focused on the greater whole. We train very bright physicians who see the tree but not the forest. In fact, not only do they see just the tree, but many see only the bark on the tree. Not only do many see just the bark on the tree, but some only the fissures on the bark on the tree, and some only see the bacteria and fungi in those fissures on the bark on the tree. In fact, many no longer even see a tree, let alone the forest.

Medical schools need to do a better job in teaching medical students about health systems thinking. Systems thinking is a holistic process and involves how complex problems can be solved through broader, team-based models of care. This is a different model than the reductionist model used in much of medical education. Reductionist thinking involves memory of facts and analysis. Holistic thinking and systems thinking requires integration and coordination. These are two totally different processes and models requiring different skills in different parts of the brain. The other thing that medical schools need to do better is to help prepare our young future physicians to work better interdependently in teams. Most physicians do not do this overly well. They are very independent, autonomous, and individualistic. This can set up a dynamic of not working easily with others and as teams. These skills of holistic, integrated, team-based, interdependent systems thinking become extremely important to tackling the complex medical issues involved in primary care.

America's medical schools are extremely valuable to our nation. They are some of the finest academic institutions in the world. The problem is that they tend to train a marvelous workforce that reinforces what academic health centers and teaching hospitals need, but fail to deliver the type of balanced workforce needed for the general service of the communities, states, and regions in which the medical schools exist. Think back to the diagram of medical care in Figure 2. The small, lower right-hand corner of boxes is where all this reductionist education and training occurs, but it only represents less than 1 percent of people's needs. It is this model that perpetuates a concentration on disease and subspecialty thinking. It is at the root of why our nation focuses on treating disease and not on promoting health.

Medical schools tend to do what they get paid to do. What they get paid to do is research with huge sums of grant money from the National Institutes of Health (NIH), and they do high-end procedures and radiology imaging for which they get large sums of financial reimbursement from Medicare and private insurance companies. This produces a mind-set in medical schools that becomes very favorable to subspecialties, proceduralists, and researchers and very toxic to primary care, community medicine, and public health. It tends to produce a workforce that's very focused on research, procedures, imaging, and reductionist subspecialties. In fact, there are 10 of the nation's medical schools that don't even have departments of family medicine, as they do not see a need to produce community physicians. So in the face of an underperforming system with the wrong type of workforce, medical schools continue to play their lyres like Nero, while the nation's health care system burns.

Business Versus Profession

American medicine is truly important to the health of our nation. Unfortunately we have gotten off track, making it more of a business than a profession. This has led to a tremendous amount of money for communities, businesses, and individuals. When $2.6 trillion per year is poured into our unaccountable health care system, there are a lot of people who are extremely well rewarded. Therefore, the energy and will to change this system is not monumentally high. Indeed, I would submit that there are 2.6 trillion reasons to have it stand just as it does for many people. Again, we have become very good at producing a back-end, reactive "sick care" system, one that is very good at doing things to people and generating large amounts of money (Figure 1). We have not been so good with the front end of the health care system, where we should more intently use the professional relationship of service to people to help improve their health. As was stated earlier, more medicine is not better medicine. In fact, it can be toxic to the patient. Our system needs to rapidly move back to its basic roots of a service-oriented profession with people at the center and away from a business and wealth-generating machine. With this basic understanding of the major problems with our health care system, let's now move into why these issues have become so important to our nation now.

Chapter 3

WHY IS OUR HEALTH CARE SYSTEM FAILING US NOW?

Let's now examine in more detail why our health care system faces major problems. What is threatening us as a nation? To do this, we must first look at what is going on both inside our country and beyond our borders.

THE WORLD IS HURTLING INTO THE INFORMATION AGE

Consider the four major ages of humanity: Hunter/Gatherer, Agricultural, Industrial, and Information. We are now progressing from the Industrial Age into the increasingly interconnected Information Age. Historically, such changes have increased productivity fiftyfold while decreasing the required workforce by 90 percent (1). Much disruptive chaos occurs because of such an increase in information flow, such large increases in productivity, and such reductions in workforce requirements; and not surprisingly, as we enter the Information Age, our country is simultaneously experiencing financial, economic, banking, educational, energy, and health care crises—along with job losses, increased unemployment, and multiple wars.

The move into the Information Age drives new ways to think, act, respond, perform business, and transfer information. As the author Thomas Friedman noted, it is making the world "flat" (2). Friedman postulates that through the Internet the world is more interconnected than ever. This is leading to more economic globalization. Because of this newly created virtual world, the geographic barriers of countries

(India, China, United States, etc.) disappear and countries begin to compete on a flat, level playing field. Information can now be instantly sent at a stroke of a key anywhere in the world. Because of the Internet, there are dynamic new ways to conduct business, compete, interact, communicate, and make money.

It is predictable that as the United States enters the Information Age, we are experiencing tremendous upheaval. We are seeing financial and economic systems in the United States, as in the rest of the industrialized world, being stressed close to the breaking point, if not in fact actually broken. Such a rapid transition into the Information Age creates much unrest and uncertainty in America's economic and financial systems, and it is not surprising that the largest single economic sector of the United States economy—health care—is undergoing major upheaval.

The Stanford economist Victor Fuchs said that it will take at least one of three conditions to cause health care to change in our country: 1) an economic depression; 2) an economic collapse or meltdown; 3) a war (3). We have all three of these things happening simultaneously. That is why the Obama administration has proactively asserted that a "crisis is a terrible thing to waste." What lies underneath a crisis is also opportunity. If a crisis can be managed well, opportunities can be produced. Indeed, when most other large nations of the world changed their health care systems, it was in such an environment. The United Kingdom, for example, made major changes in its health care system in 1947 after its economy was in shambles at the end of World War II. We now have a similar environment in our country, with changes in ways of doing business being forced by the new technologies of the Information Age. In fact, it is exactly this disruptive environment that is conducive to the innovation and changes necessary to push our health care system forward and get it unstuck. If the economy in our country was stable and things were good, there would not be the financial, the political, or the moral will to change the system. The status quo would be acceptable. Therefore a crisis is indeed a terrible thing to waste!

Having said these things, there are other reasons why we must change our health care system now. The status quo is not only unacceptable, but it is unsustainable. We have a looming crisis in our health care system that will bring our country to its knees unless we act. Let me elaborate next on why this is the case.

OUR HEALTH CARE SYSTEM COST IS UNSUSTAINABLE

The cost of our health care system is rapidly escalating. Health care as an economic engine is out of control. It has resulted in rapidly skyrocketing health insurance premiums that have shot up by 400 percent in the last 10 years, pushing the average out-of-pocket health care expenditure for every man, woman, and child in our country from approximately $4,000 per year to $7,500 per year (4). This has now risen to a projected $8,500 per year in 2012. The average monthly health insurance premium for an individual was $148 in 1990 and $402 in 2009. The average health insurance monthly premium for a family was $319 in 1990 and $1,115 in 2009 (5). According to the White House, health insurance premiums have grown four times faster than wages (6). The health care expense in our nation now exceeds $2.6 trillion per year. While this economic engine provides income and jobs for many, many people, it is drastically harming the economy of our nation, which is already struggling. The health care spending portion of the gross domestic product will grow from 17 percent to 25 percent in the year 2025, and to 50 percent in the year 2082. Not only is it affecting the nation's economy, but it is also impacting individuals' and families' financial well-being. The cost of health care now is causing a bankruptcy in America every 30 seconds (6). And if this is not enough, over 78 percent of medical bankruptcies occur with individuals who actually have health care insurance, but who are simply underinsured (7). How sad for a nation like ours that this happens daily. In fact, this is happening approximately 3,000 times a day across our country: 125 medical bankruptcies an hour, 24 hours a day, and 365 days a year.

And even for folks who are weathering this economic storm and have health care insurance, all it takes is one accident, one serious disease, one illness, a divorce, a lost job, or one stroke of bad luck and they may join the ranks of the 50 million uninsured Americans (6). The health care sector alone is not only imploding our economy today, but it will get worse going forward unless we gain control of health care costs. Health care costs are rising faster than inflation and faster than people's incomes. We must get the cost of health care under control now. Our nation has a millstone tied around our neck. That millstone is the cost of health care.

Our businesses are not faring any better. General Motors is paying more for their employees' health care than for the steel to make their cars. Starbucks is paying more for their employees' health care than it pays for its coffee. It is pressure like this on our American businesses that make them less competitive in the world marketplace. It is forcing jobs oversees, where you can pay employees less since there are no health insurance costs paid by employers for their employees. For many small businesses this is what keeps them from getting health care insurance for their workers. They simply can't afford it. The simple truth is that health care costs are holding the United States back from competing well in the globalized world market.

DEMOGRAPHIC IMPERATIVE

America is changing. Not only are we becoming more ethnically and culturally diverse as a country, we are becoming older. In the year 1900, life expectancy was 47 years. In the year 2010, life expectancy is 75.7 years for males and 80.8 years for females. If you live to be 65, then the average life span for a male is 82 years and it becomes 87 years for a female. The fastest growing population is of people over 100 years of age (8). Figure 1 below shows this large expansion of people from ages 45 to 75 that are growing older in America. Compare in this figure the increase from 2000 to 2010 in these numbers.

Figure 1. The Aging of America, Population by Age and Sex in 2000 and 2010

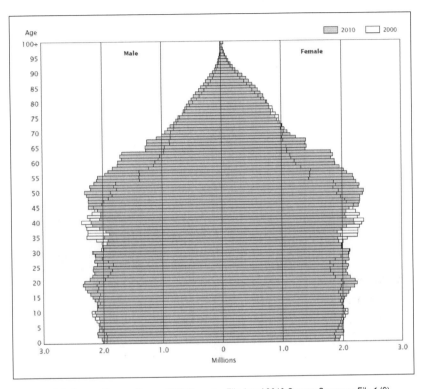

U.S. Census Bureau, *Census 2000 Summary File 1 and 2010 Census Summary File 1* (9).

Figure 2 depicts the rapid increase in the number of patients older than 85 years of age from 1900 and projected through 2050. You can see why this is becoming a rapidly growing population in our country.

Figure 2. The Aging of America, Population 85 Years Old and Above in Millions from 1900 to 2050

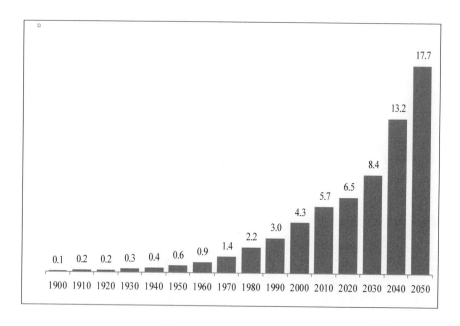

Goldstein A, Damon B. We the American ... Elderly. U.S. Department of Commerce Economics and Statistics Administration. Bureau of the Census. September 1993. [http://www.census.gov/apsd/wepeople/we-9.pdf] (10).

All of this is coupled with the fact that the number of Americans over the age of 65 will double to over 80 million the next 15 years. Approximately 40 percent of all health care expenditures in an American's entire lifetime happen in the last two years of life. In fact, chronic illness in the last two years of life accounts for 32 percent of the entire Medicare expenditure per year in our country (10). If this remains the case, the expected doubling of the Medicare population threatens an economic catastrophe. The demographic tidal wave of the aged mandates that we get on top of major health care reform now. As I mentioned in Chapter 2, Medicare is programmed to become insolvent fiscally in 2024, just at the same time that we have large numbers of Medicare patients crashing into our health care system.

AMERICA IS NO LONGER A WORLD LEADER IN HEALTH OUTCOMES

Despite the amount of money being spent on health care, there is a major disconnect in this improving the health of our nation. In fact, there is a major distinction between health care and health. Health care is a process where the health care system interacts with people. It represents all the services and the total amount of money that is spent in our health care system. Ideally, health care is a means to an end. The end should be health. The problem is that what health care is generating for the nation's health is not directly proportional to health outcomes. We spend 40 percent more on health care in our country than the next closest country, which is Switzerland (11). However, what we get for this is mediocre health outcomes at best. In fact, America is going backwards and farther down the list of health outcomes. According to the World Health Organization, we rank 37th in the world for our health care outcomes (12). According to the Commonwealth Fund, of the 19 nations surveyed, we are 19th out of 19 in our nation's health (13). Not only are we 19th of 19, but our ranking fell from 15th to 19th from 2006 to 2008 (13).

This is embarrassing for a nation as rich, progressive, and creative as ours. We have a significant discrepancy between how we spend money on health care and its relationship to health. We are spending our money on the wrong things. Instead of spending on health promotion, wellness, prevention, and chronic disease management on the front end of health care, we are spending our dollars on disease, illness, high-end procedures, and imaging on the back end of health care. Instead of spending pennies on the dollar to treat, control, or prevent hypertension, diabetes, heart attacks, strokes, and kidney failure, we are spending tens of thousands of dollars on the back end of health care for heart attacks, strokes, and renal dialysis. Instead of being proactive about health, we are being reactive about health care. This is why, despite the massive amounts of money we pump into our health care system, we can only generate second-rate outcomes for our nation's health. Our nation's health care system has become more enraptured with generating wealth than on generating health.

WE HAVE INCONSISTENT INSURANCE COVERAGE

Another reason why now is the time to change our health care system is that we have a rising number of uninsured people. We have more and more people who are struggling to afford basic health insurance. As the number of uninsured now climbs over 50 million, which represents approximately 17 percent of our population, the number of have-nots in the system is growing. We do have a large number of people with the means to get health care whenever they need it. In fact, our system is excellent at having an MRI or a CAT scan done tomorrow if you have means to see a physician and insurance or personal money to pay for those tests. However, if you do not have health insurance coverage or money to gain timely access to the system, then you live sicker and you die younger. Studies have been very clear on this fact (14). The uninsured, underinsured, poor, and ethnically and educationally disadvantaged do not have similar access to timely, high-quality care and therefore have poorer health outcomes than the well-insured, richer, better-educated, and predominantly white members of society.

Part of what is causing the United States to have poor health care outcomes is the lack of basic health care insurance for a large percentage of our population. In fact, if you take a look at both the uninsured and the underinsured, this represents approximately 75 million adults, which is 42 percent of all adults aged 19 to 64 (13). It is when we combine health outcomes of those with means and those without, that we see our ranking against other nations drop. That is why expanding meaningful health insurance coverage becomes a major imperative. This will allow people to have the basic health care coverage they need, when they need it, to maximize their health. Allowing people to be seen by the right health care provider, at the right time, in the right place, for the right reasons becomes important to optimizing health.

We see health care disparities in our country among different socioeconomic classes partly due to the fact that these groups have lower rates of insurance and fewer sources of usual care. Their lower socioeconomic position in our society locks them into the have-not category of receiving health care. If you have basic health insurance and a usual source of care, your health is better (15). If you lack health insurance coverage and a usual source of care, then your health is poorer. This leads to the disparities we see in health care in our country for such conditions as colon cancer, cervical cancer, heart attacks, strokes, and heart failure (16, 17). This is why meaningful health insurance coverage must improve.

WE STUMBLE WITH LACKLUSTER HEALTH INFORMATION TECHNOLOGY (HIT)

Our nation operates an unregulated, non-standardized free-for-all of fragmented, nonintegrated health care information systems. Other industrialized nations have moved much faster and more successfully than we have in their adoption of electronic medical records. This is yet another reason why we need health care transformation now to correct this disarray and enable our country to move forward. Abraham Lincoln did many wonderful things for our country, in addition to leading us through our own Civil War. One of the little recognized things that Lincoln did was to integrate the railroad system. In 1862 we had three gauge widths of rail track. This made it impossible to have one nationalized rail system used by trains or train companies with varied widths of wheels. Lincoln standardized the rail gauge width to 48 inches. This decision then allowed all trains to build for a common standard which interlinked and opened up all of America to easier rail travel (18). This did not come easy, I am sure, to the railroad companies that needed to change their trains and their wheelbase sizes. It also created much work and costs to tear out the wrong-sized rail track for the newly standardized rail track width. However, it was the right thing to do for the good of our country. We face a similar dilemma now in our health information technologies and our electronic medical record systems. Currently there are many systems and programs being utilized that do not talk to each other. The federal government must step forward and standardize the interoperability of information systems and electronic medical record utilization so that we have a seamless system that easily moves information from one office to another over a standard system. We must develop a single gauge rail of operability for our electronic medical records. Surprisingly, this standardization does not exist in American medicine.

Part of the benefit of transforming our health care system is to incorporate the advancements of health information technology and the electronic medical record into better ways of exchanging information between physicians, hospitals, emergency rooms, clinics, community health care agencies, and other systems of health care. Health information technology (HIT) represents all of the electronic equipment needed to gather, coordinate, tabulate, compare, analyze, integrate, and communicate health care information from point A to point B. The electronic medical record (EMR) is a subset of HIT and represents a computer that stores and retrieves data on a patient in a secure manner that guarantees privacy. It essentially does away with paper records. Paper is often ineffective, with jumbled records and barriers to finding information when you need it. When you can find information in the paper record, it is often illegible. This has led to the notion that "paper kills." Often important pieces of information are missing or misfiled in the paper record, leading others who are dependent on that timely piece of information to overlook it when important decisions are being made about people's lives and health.

You would think that more of medicine would be using HIT and EMRs. The truth is that approximately 20.5 percent of physician's offices use EMRs (19). Only about 45 percent of emergency rooms use EMRs (20). Only about 34 percent of hospitals use EMRs (21). This lack of HIT and EMRs, as well as other systems-related health care issues, leads to about 100,000 unnecessary medical deaths from mistakes each year in the United States (22). The United States lags behind most of the industrialized nations in EMR adoption (23).

Why does the American health care system struggle with

electronic medical records and other information systems? There is one simple reason for this. The American health care system pays for health care regardless of how it is recorded. It does not matter at this point in time if this information is recorded in written form or electronically. Since the average cost per physician is $75,000 to install an electronic medical record, there is little incentive to do so (24). In any other economic sector, other than health care, if there is new technology introduced into that sector, those costs are passed on to the customer. That does not happen in medicine. The billing for health care costs are fixed and set by Medicare, Medicaid, and private insurance companies. Therefore, you can only bill a designated amount for that service. There is no differential payment for that service being provided by an electronic medical record or not. Hence, with no increased incentive financially, this is not something most physicians feel compelled to do. In fact, many have told me there is no way they will invest the time, energy, money, and resources to make this change unless there are financial incentives to do so. To boost this use, there must be built in a differential fee, perhaps as little as several dollars extra for visits done electronically versus being recorded on paper. It only stands to reason that, if appropriately paid for, the use of computerized billing and records systems will increase. These changes need to happen to maximize the efficiency, accuracy, and quality of our United States health care system.

WE HAVE A PRIMARY CARE CRISIS

The generation of our primary care workforce in this nation is in a crisis mode. We are not generating enough primary care physicians. We will not have timely, accessible health care for the people of this country unless we fix this problem starting now. It takes seven years to produce a primary care physician. This process takes four years of medical school and three years of residency training to become a family physician, a general internist, or a general pediatrician. That pipeline of seven years is a long road. If we increase and expand health care coverage, as was discussed above, but we do not have the right workforce to see all of these patients, then we will only exacerbate our problems.

The state of Massachusetts has taught us this lesson. In 2006, the progressive Massachusetts legislature expanded health care coverage to 97.6 percent of the Massachusetts citizenry (25). Although an unprecedented number of people now had health care coverage, what the Commonwealth of Massachusetts uncovered was that there were not enough primary care providers to deliver this type of care. Therefore, Massachusetts experienced a persistent problem with access to care, with an increase in waiting times to see a primary care physician reaching 47 to 50 days, resulting in an increase in ER utilization and cost to the health care system (26). That is why as we move forward with health care reform, we must immediately work to rebalance the health care workforce. Health care insurance coverage alone does not equal health. Unless we have an adequate number of the right types of physicians to deliver front-end health care to the system, we will not achieve the best health for our people.

The health care workforce balance in countries outside of the United States is about 50 percent of the workforce in primary care and 50 percent in subspecialties (27). In our country, that balance today is 70 percent in subspecialties and 30 percent in primary care (28), and this unbalance is becoming worse. In the last 10 years, medical school graduates have chosen to go into subspecialties at the rate of 90 percent (29). This, coupled with the retirement of many primary care physicians over the next 10 years, will only compound the workforce crisis. Sadly, this is not a new problem for America. This crisis in primary care and the extinction of the generalist physician and family physician in favor of subspecialist physicians has been happening for a long time. In fact, there has been a steady decline in the percentage of primary care physicians in the United States from 40.2 percent of the total number of physicians in 1970 to 32.6 percent in 2006 (30).

As early as 1933, the *Journal of the American Medical Association* noted that "the overgrowth of specialism now [was] so bitterly complained of, and the fadeout of the general practitioner [was occurring]." (31) In 1949, Stanley R. Truman, MD, president-elect of the American Academy of General Practitioners (AAGP), now the American Academy of Family Physicians (AAFP), stated, "Too many specialists are as dangerous to the quality and quantity of medical care in a community as too few." (32) In 1948 Eugene Smith, writing for *Life* magazine, chronicled the week in the life of Doctor Ernest Ceriani, a rural general practitioner in Kremmling, Colorado, a town located 115 miles west of Denver and at that time contained 1,000 people and the surrounding 400 square miles contained 1,000 more people that he cared for. Dr. Ceriani was the lone country doctor, known as the "G.P." and served as the physician, surgeon, obstetrician, pediatrician, psychiatrist, dentist, oculist, and laboratory technician to them all. Dr. Ceriani could care for all but one case in every 100 patients. Kremmling, Colorado was lucky to have Dr. Ceriani. But countless communities at that time did not have such a physician. Not even one. In 1948, the nation's medical schools were sending the majority of their graduates into specialization. Two things were felt necessary to reverse that trend. First, there was a call for medical school reform, away from portraying specialization as a glamorous occupation and general practice as just the thankless chore of a drudge (33). The second obstacle identified was the need for small communities to make an effort to attract general practitioners to the community. This condition in the 1930s and 1940s frustratingly continued unchanged as time rolled on. In fact, it only worsened. For example, the Citizens Commission on Graduate Medical Education observed in 1966 that "specialization has been accompanied by an alarming decline in the number of physicians who devote themselves to continuing and comprehensive care of the whole individual." (34)

Unfortunately, our nation has still not made headway on this problem. Over-specialization of the medical workforce at the dire expense of the generalist physician/primary care family physician workforce has steadily worsened over the last eight decades. Primary care remains in crisis. To rectify this, America needs an overhaul of our entire health care system to one that values and respects what primary care physicians mean to their patients and communities. This must be reflected in better payment for primary care physicians so that students do not choose a subspecialty over primary care for financial reasons. We must also unburden the primary care physician from much of his or her administrative paperwork so that they can devote more of their time to caring for their patients and their communities. America's medical schools must step up to the plate as well and retarget their efforts on training more primary care physicians for the many communities that need them. Every patient and every community like Kremmling, Colorado, needs a Dr. Ceriani. In fact, they need a small, dedicated team of one to two doctors, one to two mid-level practitioners (such as a nurse practitioner or physician assistant), and several nurses or medical assistants working as a team to provide sustainable, ongoing, comprehensive, and continuous care to the community. This is a priority in the Affordable Care Act reform law, because without a strong backbone of primary care, you have nothing to build a health care system on.

WE DON'T DEFINE PRIMARY CARE AS AN INTEGRATED TEAM

Care providers in our health care system are more known for fighting with each other than working with each other. Unfortunately, there is a lot of infighting in medicine among different types of physicians; physicians and nurses; physicians, nurses, and administrators; and just about everyone else you can imagine. A key feature of primary care is that it is a team endeavor. As we go forward, we must work closely with our nurse practitioner and physician assistant colleagues to help expand the funnel of the undersized and undermanned primary care workforce. These skilled health care providers must complement the primary care workforce to amplify the number that serve the front end of health care. These providers will help in the short term, and definitely will help in the long term, as we build a better-balanced health care system.

Part of the problem, however, is that the same forces that lure medical students to subspecialize rather than to go into primary care are also causing nurse practitioners and physician assistants to subspecialize. They are also following the money, the status, and the lifestyle. Even though the purpose of creating nurse practitioners and physician assistants (PAs) in the first place was to augment the primary care workforce in the mid-1960s when these programs were created, we are now seeing the payment system steer these providers into the more highly paid and lucrative subspecialties. This is a problem that must be corrected if we are to create the workforce we need rather than the workforce we have: a workforce of intent and not a workforce by default.

Some advocate the idea that nurse practitioners or physician assistants are equivalent to, or even replace, primary care physicians (35). This movement will have major difficulty for two very important reasons. The first is that there are large differences in each group's training. Training a nurse practitioner or physician assistant requires basically 500 to 1,000 hours of clinical training on top of a bachelor's degree (36). Training a primary care physician after his or her bachelor's degree requires four years of medical school (representing about 4,000 hours of clinical work in addition to classroom work) to first become a physician, and then an additional 10,000 hours of training to complete a three-year residency in family medicine, general internal medicine, or general pediatrics. The knowledge depth, the broad scope of practice, the comprehensive integration of training, and the ability to perform a wide spectrum of invasive procedures thus requires approximately 14,000 hours of training for a physician. This is markedly different than the time necessary to train a nurse practitioner or physician assistant and results in much broader, comprehensive, and complete skills.

Please do not get me wrong. Nurse practitioners and physician assistants are highly valued members of the team. However, they are not substitutes for primary care physicians. The function of the primary care physician in leading an integrated team is not because of some desire for control. It is because of accountability and responsibility. A comprehensive depth of knowledge and training allows the primary care physician to naturally pilot this broad health care team. The myth that nurse practitioners and physician assistants are similar and equal in training to primary care physicians is simply not true and must be abandoned. This disappointingly is a myth that is also being propagated by some physicians and some medical schools to dissuade medical students from choosing to go into primary care. At a time when we need primary care physicians the most, we have forces working in counter-productive ways.

The second reason that nurse practitioners and physician assistants are touted as possible replacements for primary care physicians is a more insidious and dangerous one. There are some in the health care industry who believe that nurse practitioners and physician assistants should be generic replacements for the entire front end of the health care system. An underlying motive in asserting this comes from a desire to perpetuate the status quo of our broken health care system. If nurse practitioners and physician assistants by training care for fewer types of comprehensive problems at the front end of the health care system, then they will refer more patients than do primary care physicians to subspecialty physicians, the emergency rooms, and into the hospitals. You see, if primary care physicians do the job they are trained to do, it means much less work downstream in the form of consultations, labs, procedures, emergency room visits, and hospitalizations for the rest of the health care system. This is why it is important to not lose primary care physicians from our workforce if we truly want to reform our health care system. Their comprehensive skills are invaluable. The plan should be to have nurse practitioners and physician assistants working with primary care physicians as part of integrated teams, not working separately from them. By doing this we further strengthen the primary care team. We must act now, using an all-inclusive approach on this primary care workforce crisis. We need to unite the primary care team, not leave it divided and fractured. I have become fond of an adage I heard from one of my dear Canadian family medicine colleagues, who argued that every patient deserves a family physician *and* a nurse, not a family physician *or* a nurse. We must all learn to work better together and to act as a team.

WE MISUNDERSTAND THE IMPORTANCE OF RELATIONSHIPS AND END-OF-LIFE ISSUES

As was mentioned earlier, we will have a doubling of the Medicare population from 40 plus million to over 80 million people in the next 15 years. Fifteen years! This will bring with it a lot of downstream deliberations on the nature of death itself. Forty percent of all health care costs in one's life come in the person's last two years of life. Forty percent! Primary care is critical to health care reform, in part because this is where major interactions with patients often occur about important end-of-life considerations. Primary care must be the front door of health care. It is where the relationship between the physician and the patient is forged. It is through this interaction that a trusting relationship is built. Once built, this relationship is what reinforces education, knowledge, shared responsibilities, and compliance. A patient does not care how much his or her physician knows until they know how much the physician cares. Only after a trusted relationship is established and the patient knows that the physician is there for them in a caring, non-judgmental manner will they believe them and follow their advice, guidance, and recommendations. It is in this relationship that shared plans and mutual responsibilities occur, leading to a patient's compliance with his or her health care plan. My relationships with my patients are more important than any medications I will ever prescribe for them or any procedures that will ever be done for them. The stronger the relationship, the better the patient's satisfaction and willingness to work with their physician on the multifaceted issues that define the patient's health. This interface between the physician and the patient can be appreciated in the figure below.

Figure 3. The Importance of the Primary Care Physician–Patient Relationship

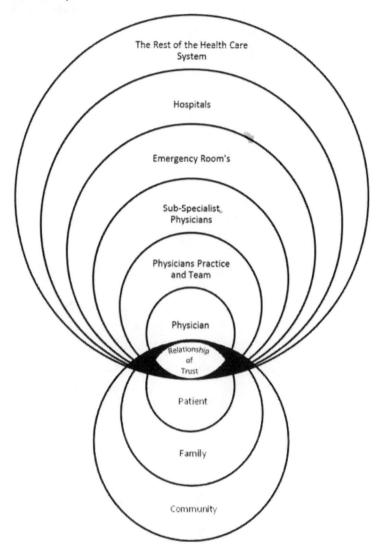

The Rest of the Health Care System

Hospitals

Emergency Room's

Sub-Specialist Physicians

Physicians Practice and Team

Physician

Relationship of Trust

Patient

Family

Community

It is through a trusted relationship with primary care physicians, nurse practitioners, physician assistants, and nurses that people are guided through the complexity of health care. Headway on health happens through primary care. This holds true for all phases of care, from acute and urgent care to chronic ongoing disease management, preventive health maintenance, and end-of-life health care management. Within this deep, trusted relationship, meaningful discussions about end-of-life treatment and care can best unfold. Through these conversations, choices and options can be considered and discussed with patients and families. By sensitively and compassionately dealing with the patient and his or her personal values, the physician can explore options and end-of-life desires. An entire armada of health care options can be lined up if the patient so desires, or the patient can meaningfully and knowledgeably decide that they do not want nor expect that everything will be done for them to sustain life. In the absence of this end-of-life information, the health care system will err on the side of doing everything to keep the patient alive. This discussion is not to ration care; this is to not deny care, but by discussing the *patient's* wants and expectations at the end of life their wishes can be carried out. In a health care system of unlimited possibilities, a discussion must be held about what are the realistic considerations. End-of-life choices are unique for each patient and family, and can only be sorted out one patient and one family at a time through the care and compassion of the patient's trusted personal physician. These are not "death panels" as they were branded in the 2009–2010 health care debates. If these discussions do not clearly occur then costs can run up exorbitantly, for very little or no return to the patient's life expectancy or quality of that remaining life.

When my time comes and I am lying on my deathbed, I want to be in my home, warm, dry, and surrounded by people I love. I want to be free of as much pain and anxiety as possible. What I do not want is to be in a hospital intensive care unit hooked up to monitors, and have intravenous lines in three areas of my body and tubes in most of my body orifices. I don't want buzzers and alarms and the metronome of my heart beat beeping to all within 10 yards. I don't want to be surrounded by those who don't know me. I want simplicity and quiet. I don't want chaos and noise. I want to die in peace and with dignity.

This is why having a deep bond with your physician and their team is essential.

Unfortunately, this concept was taken out of context and spun into the boogeyman of "death panels" and "rationing of care." Instead of recognizing the necessity for physicians to provide sensitivity and skill in a complex, caring discussion about end-of-life concerns, it was categorized by the opponents of health care reform as the creation of sinister death panels waiting to pull the plug on grandma's life. These are not death panel discussions but realistic, end-of-life discussions where each individual person's beliefs, values, and requests are understood, honored, and followed by the family, the physician, and the health care team. This is the value of the primary care physician and the relationship that can only be built with time. The primary care physician's broad scope of knowledge in all areas of medicine provides insight and perspective. It is formed on the basis of many prior visits that builds a richness and context of shared decisions that now lead to decisions of what defines a lifetime for the patient.

If we now reflect on the primary care physician and the importance of the doctor–patient relationship to the 80 plus million Medicare-aged patients that are moving through life, you can see that we have a tremendous challenge ahead in having the right primary care physicians to build these relationships and have these discussions. Subspecialist physicians can have these discussions, but typically do not have the richness of the relationship or the continuity of time with the patient. As a result, they often lack the comprehensive knowledge needed to deal with all the complexities involved in these discussions. Not because these subspecialist physicians aren't capable to have these discussions, but because they don't have the breadth of knowledge of the patient, let alone the patient's family. Our health care system often defaults to decisions made by physicians who don't really know the patient. This is not ideal for the patient or for the health care system. Without this knowledge, without this relationship, the robotic response is simply to do more. It is easier to do more than to do less, because not only will our health care system pay for more, but because it is then easier to evade an end-of-life discussion.

Without facing these important decisions, the roaring engine of health care will just churn onward, at the detriment to the entire American economy. It is only through managing the tangled issues of health and the thorny issues around death that we can start to impact health care costs. These sensitive discussions should be done with the physician who best knows the patient. This is why the primary care crisis is an important one; one that must be fixed. Without such a remedy, the United States will not have the right types of physicians to deal with the kinds of issues that surround the front end of health care and end-of-life care. Where is Dr. Ceriani when we need him?

Chapter 4

AMERICA'S HISTORY OF HEALTH CARE REFORM

Ben Franklin once said, "The farther back you look, the farther forward you see." Let's review a short history of our nation's struggle to transform the United States health care system from its traditional medical approach—an approach often reactive and absorbed primarily in treating sickness—to a system that in contrast would proactively and aggressively pursue health. What attempts have we made in the past to foster such a transformation, and how successful have we been? More importantly, how have we dealt with a most fundamental question: is health care a basic American right or a money-based privilege?

The first attempts to change our health care system started in 1911 with Teddy Roosevelt when he ran for president on a platform calling for health care reform of an unregulated, chaotic, uncoordinated medical industry that would better serve and assist businesses of the time (1). Since then there have been 11 presidents who have tackled this daunting issue, including Franklin D. Roosevelt, Harry Truman, John F. Kennedy, Lyndon B. Johnson, Richard Nixon, Gerald Ford, Jimmy Carter, George H.W. Bush, Bill Clinton, George W. Bush, and Barack Obama (see Table 1).

Table 1. A Brief Time Table of Health Care Reform Efforts

1910	Flexner Report was released on medical education in the United States and Canada
1911–1912	Teddy Roosevelt advocated for health insurance reform for businesses
1915	Several states attempted a state-based system of mandatory health insurance
1920	Proposed voluntary insurance and group medicine—"socialized medicine"

1929	Great Depression aggravated the people's need for health care support
1935	Social Security Act passed as part of the New Deal by Franklin D. Roosevelt; health care reform pulled out
1938	Further efforts for health care reform blocked by Congress
1945	President Truman attempted to pass National Health Insurance (Fair Deal)
1946	Hill-Burton Act, which called for hospital construction and expansion, was passed
1947	United Kingdom adopted a Nationalized Health Care System
1948	Truman reattempted to pass National Health Insurance
1949	Opposition from the AMA, Southern Democrats, and eroding public support killed health care reform efforts
1954	Employers' contributions to health benefits became tax-exempt
1965	Medicare and Medicaid signed into law by Lyndon B. Johnson
1972	Health Security Act as a Universal Single-Payer Plan was proposed by Senator Ted Kennedy
1974	Dueling National Health Insurance plans proposed by President Richard Nixon and Senator Ted Kennedy were killed by the Watergate scandal
1977–1980	Congress rejected cost control efforts by President Carter and National Health Insurance by Senator Ted Kennedy
1983	Medicare Prospective Payment System—a charge-based system changed to a fixed payment based upon the patient's diagnosis
1991	President George H.W. Bush promoted health care tax credits and purchasing pools
1993	Health Security Act proposed by President and First Lady Clinton—managed competition
1995–2000	Managed care attempted to control costs
1997	Children's Health Insurance Program (CHIP)
1997	Balance Budget Reduction Act (BBRA) with the imposition of the Medicare Sustainable Growth Rate (SGR) formula
2003	Medicare Modernization Act (MMA), Medicare prescription drug bill
2009–2010	Current efforts of the 111th Congress and the Obama administration at health reform
March 23, 2010	The Patient Protection and Affordable Care Act (PPACA) was signed into law by President Obama, becoming Public Law 111-48; the largest reform of health care since Medicare and Medicaid in 1965
2010–2012	Congressional Democrats and Republicans and President Obama struggled to right-size health care reform

Almost all presidents since FDR—including both Democrats and Republicans—have had some role in shaping our health care system, reinforcing the idea that health care reform for the good of our nation is not a Democratic nor a Republican issue, but an American issue.

Prior to the first health care reform efforts in 1911, there wasn't much of a system to reform. Science was not advanced enough to influence medicine and very few medications had any significant value. After the turn of the century, public and preventive health efforts, vaccinations, water purification, hand washing, good hygiene, and other ways to prevent infections started to gain a scientific foothold. These advances started making differences in morbidity and mortality in people's lives. In 1910 Abraham Flexner produced his report on the status of our nation's medical schools (2). This report critically identified poor-quality education in many medical schools and the unregulated training of physicians. As a result, many medical schools closed and a structured medical education curriculum was developed. This report is what became responsible for the development of a centralized hospital-based medical education program over a more balanced community-based alternative.

The year 1915 saw efforts at state-based systems of mandatory health insurance. In 1920, the term "socialized medicine" was born with proposals for voluntary insurance and group medicine (1). There were attempts in the 1920s and '30s at some sort of health insurance so that people could at least afford basic health insurance coverage and receive help with the expenses of hospitalizations or surgeries if needed. Prior to that time people with means could pay for these things to be done, but people without means would either get no care or could become bankrupt by receiving it.

These ideas became more profound as America sank into the Great Depression from 1929 to 1939. Franklin D. Roosevelt tried to incorporate a national health insurance plan along with his legislation to create the Social Security Act. However, there was major push back from physician groups as they did not want to see government regulate the practice of medicine or fix health care costs. They believed that a free market and patient choice should be the purview of doctors and hospitals and not of the federal government, and national health care insurance for all was taken out of the Social Security Act that was passed during FDR's tenure in 1935.

Roosevelt wanted to get back to national health insurance, but by 1938 Congress was no longer supportive. During this time (and as early as 1914), employers were also looking for some sort of insurance benefits for their workers. This movement was somewhat sporadic, but the idea of expanding coverage as a benefit to workers and as a competitive enticement for them to work for certain companies was gaining traction. Now, let's consider several noteworthy efforts to provide health care coverage to Americans that stand out since FDR's time.

NATIONALIZED HEALTH INSURANCE

President Truman in 1945 again proposed national health insurance in which the federal government would provide for all Americans. This proposed system would not control the doctors or hospitals, but it would pay all of the bills by means of a national single-payer system. At the end of World War II a euphoria existed in our country and the political will was in place for Truman to try again to do what FDR had been unsuccessful in achieving. In his address to Congress in November of 1945, President Truman stated, "In the past the benefits of modern medical science have not been enjoyed by our citizens with any degree of equality. Nor are they today. Nor will they be in the future unless government is bold enough to do something about it. We should resolve now that the health of this nation is a national concern; that financial barriers in the way of attaining health shall be removed; that the health of all of its citizens deserves the help of all the nation." (3) These were bold words in a pivotal time of change following World War II, and 75 percent of the country supported national health insurance (4). However, the same forces that sunk FDR's plan of health care reform reemerged. Physician organizations and insurance organizations saw this again as price fixing, government control, the creation of a welfare state, and the movement toward a totalitarian socialist state. During this time communism was spreading from the Soviet Union to its neighboring countries, as well as China. These fears flamed into the mantra that America does not want "socialized medicine." These forces prevailed, and America lost its momentum to push for a nationalized health care system.

At the same time in the United Kingdom the exact same movement was playing out, but with a drastically different outcome. The United Kingdom adopted a nationalized health care system for its entire population in 1947. Why did the United Kingdom do this and the United States not? What were the differences between those two countries at that time? The opportunity existed in both countries. One stepped forward. The other did not. These differences in our countries' culture and mind-set will be more fully explored in Chapters 5 and 6. The United Kingdom was in shambles after the war. Its economy was struggling. The creation of a nationalized health care system was a way to unite its people around a common cause. It was something the country could focus on for the common good. The United States by contrast was not in shambles. Other than Pearl Harbor, we had not been bombed. Our cities were not in ruin. Our economy was a robust, wartime economy and doing extremely well. The nation had been beefed up by the war and its resulting "military-industrial complex" was leading to newfound prosperity. The level of pain and suffering was in no way as great. Health care reform was not needed to bring a nation together, and in some camps and corners, not wanted. Instead of healthcare reform being seen as a basic good, it was seen as a forced evil.

With the difference of these two countries' ethos in mind, Truman, upon his surprise reelection in 1948, again attempted to transform America's health care system into a nationalized health care system. Unfortunately, the same forces that sunk this plan earlier again stonewalled progress. Because of this opposition, the view of the American public on bills to transform our health care system declined from 75 percent in support several years earlier to only 21 percent in support for these later reform efforts (5). Health care reform in the form of Nationalized Health Insurance at this point in our nation's history was basically over.

THE RISE OF PRIVATE COMMUNITY RATED HEALTH INSURANCE

As was noted earlier, the concept of workers health insurance emerged after Teddy Roosevelt's time in 1914 and gained momentum as a private sector phenomenon. The people of the era did not want to see our federal government become the source of health care and so the private system became the entity that resonated most with the spirit of America's capitalistic, free-enterprise system. During the time of the late 1940s and 1950s, Blue Cross and Blue Shield were highly respected companies that worked off of the concept of *community rating*. This included having as many people as possible in the pool so that premiums and costs could be shared equally by all. Therefore, premiums were the same for the young and the old, the diseased and the infirmed, and the benefits were the same for all. It was under this concept of community rating that the money could be spread to include as much coverage as possible. Of course what comes with that concept is that the young, healthy individuals are relatively overcharged to help make up for the elderly and sick individuals who are relatively undercharged. This concept was felt to be important, however, because the elderly and the sick were not in a position to afford a higher-priced insurance. The cost was spread to all for the good of all. The young, strong, and healthy would help those who were not. A sense of solidarity had emerged in those early days of community rating that seemed to value the whole greater than it did the individuals in the system.

THE RISE OF FOR-PROFIT EXPERIENCE RATED INSURANCE

Several years after Blue Cross and Blue Shield were doing much to expand coverage and insurance for as many as possible, for-profit insurance companies started to emerge. They recognized that in this marketplace there was money to be made by subdividing age groups, disease entities, and risk pools. They moved from the concept of *community rating* to one of *experience rating*. This basically provided the concept that a person's premium would be based on their age and risk factors and their prior year's utilization of the health care system. Of course this led to lower premiums and costs for the young and healthy, and higher cost premiums for the elderly and the sick. These health insurance companies were very good at segmenting the marketplace and using actuarial data to drive premiums. This was a very successful business model and made a lot of money for these health insurance companies. Unfortunately, it left many people with preexisting problems and diseases, and the aged, in a very precarious position. The emergence of for-profit, experience-rated health insurance became a regressive step away from the whole and started to refocus on the individual. Instead of being about "us" it became more about "me." In addition to this rapid growth of health insurance companies, employers' contributions to health benefits became tax-exempt in 1954, leading to the rapid expansion of employer-based health coverage through these health insurance companies. Health insurance benefits were seen as a tool to lure workers to a company as well as a tool to retain them.

MEDICARE AND MEDICAID

As can be readily appreciated, we moved quickly back to a diverging have versus have-not system. Those with means could access employer health insurance or buy their own, but those without means—the poor, disabled, sick, infirmed, or elderly—struggled to get health care. Even if they could get it, it was expensive and many were forced out of receiving basic health care. This led to a continuing debate on what our society should do for those without means, most notably the elderly and the poor. Kennedy, as early as 1960, spoke to this issue as he ran for president. Public support grew for a broader plan now known as "Medicare" and 69 percent of America favored it in 1962 (6). For this reason, President Kennedy favored legislation that was being crafted to create such a plan. Unfortunately, with President Kennedy's assassination America lost a major champion for health care reform. But Lyndon B. Johnson felt obligated to push on with President Kennedy's plan. This was reminiscent of Truman following up on his mentor Franklin D. Roosevelt's proposals. In 1964, President Johnson was swept into office along with strong Democratic majorities in the House and Senate and in 1965 Medicare and Medicaid were created to help the have-nots in Johnson's "Great Society." However, the American Medical Association, some insurance companies, the American Hospital Association, and other organizations vigorously fought Johnson's measures. Their overwhelming concern was again fear of taking America down a "socialized" or "communistic" track by a "massive governmental intervention" on price fixing, while at the same time intruding on the sacred doctor–patient relationship. Even with such opposition, however, there was a growing public need to ensure that the elderly, the poor, and the disabled had health care security. The American Hospital Association and some of the private insurance companies in the end broke with the American Medical Association and supported the proposed legislation. On July 30, 1965 the Medicare and Medicaid law was signed into existence, becoming the largest single governmental expansion of health care in the history of our country (1, 7). Upon signing the bill, President Johnson said, "No longer will older Americans be denied the healing miracles of modern medicine. No longer will illness crush and destroy the savings they have so carefully put away over a lifetime so that they might enjoy dignity in their later years. No longer will young families see their own incomes, and their own hopes, eaten away simply because they are carrying out their deep moral obligations to their parents, and to their uncles, and their aunts." (8) To honor Truman for his dedicated work on this issue 20 years earlier, President Johnson went to the Truman Library in Independence, Missouri, where President Truman sat next to President Johnson and witnessed him sign Medicare and Medicaid into law.

COMPETING NATIONAL HEALTH PLANS OF THE EARLY 1970S

However, there were still issues of coverage, access, and cost of health care. In response to this, Senator Ted Kennedy proposed a single-payer National Health Insurance plan in the early 1970s. Not to be outdone, Republican President Nixon introduced his Comprehensive Health Insurance Plan (CHIP) in 1974, aimed at building a comprehensive private sector insurance plan to meet the issues of cost, coverage, and access. In the spring of 1974 there was bipartisan support for health care reform; nobody in Congress wanted to be seen as obstructionist (1). The issue revolved around a single payer government run system versus a private health insurance system. We stood very close as a nation to passing further comprehensive health care reform at that moment. The American Medical Association continued to be opposed but no longer could it use the argument of "socialized medicine" for this Comprehensive Health Insurance Plan was supported by President Nixon, a strong, outspoken anti-communist. However, Watergate intervened and all forward momentum on health care reform abruptly stopped. Senator Kennedy later lamented that it was a mistake for him to not have supported the Nixon proposal because that was a moment in which further reform could have been accomplished (9). President Ford attempted to resurrect this legislation in 1974 and 1975 after President Nixon resigned, but by then further interest on health care reform was moribund.

THE LATE 1970S

When Jimmy Carter became president, he narrowed his focus to cost control, especially at the hospital level. This was after pledging support for national health insurance in his campaign, and Senator Kennedy took him to task over this change in position. Kennedy drafted another bill focusing on private insurance companies, in which they would compete for customers using insurance cards. These cards would be paid for mostly by employers for their employees and by the government for the elderly and poor. After three years of work these bills never made it through Congress (10).

THE CLINTON ERA

Growing out of the George H.W. Bush presidency of the late '80s and early '90s was a 1991 health care plan that would have controlled costs through tax credits, subsidies, and purchasing pools. This plan didn't catch on, however, and with the election of Bill Clinton came a new shot at major comprehensive health care reform. Clinton wanted to make massive changes to the health care system to expand coverage, increase quality, control costs, and provide health care for all. This plan was called the Health Security Act. Clinton was labeled as a tax-and-spend Democrat by opponents, and he morphed his thinking into a plan of "managed competition" to garner broader support. This concept was a hybridization of both progressive and conservative thoughts. This plan would have physicians, insurance companies, and other organizations compete to provide health care plans to pooled alliances of employers and individuals. The plan was designed to control costs through competition, improve quality, provide expanded universal coverage, impose individual and employer mandates, and create health purchasing alliances and a health security card. Although the president and First Lady Hilary Clinton sought to strike the right balance, the process they used eventually sunk this plan. They gathered many experts behind closed doors and came up with a very complex health care plan of over 1,400 pages. There was no major involvement by many major organizations of the time, including the American Medical Association, American Hospital Association, American Health Insurance Plans, pharmaceutical companies, device manufacturers, members of Congress, big and small business groups, and consumer groups. As a result there was very little organized support for the Clinton plan. Once it was rolled out it was lambasted by all of these groups as being too complex, too costly, and bad for America. While this plan was effectively opposed and organizations lobbied actively against it, the divided Democratic majority in Congress could not gain enough votes to pass the bill.

Former President James Madison once said, "We are not a government. We are a nation of special interests that run our government." These special interests rallied and sunk the Clinton health care plan. The lesson learned from the Clinton approach was that all stakeholders need to be brought to the table. If they are not present and do not have some say and ownership in the process, then they will become part of its destruction and not part the solution.

In 1997 President Clinton, however, was successful in getting a Republican Congress with bipartisan agreement to expand Medicaid coverage to more low-income children through the Children's Health Insurance Program (CHIP, though not to be confused with Nixon's Comprehensive Health Insurance Plan). Also in that year, the Balanced Budget Reduction Act (BBRA) sought to control the wildly escalating costs of Medicare spending by implementing a draconian sustainable growth rate formula (SGR) that would attempt to control Medicare costs. This law in essence cut physicians' pay based upon Medicare spending that exceeded spending targets. Although this formula was initially successful, it led to eight years of annual, special congressional legislation to freeze the cuts to physicians. The reason for the freeze was that the American Medical Association and other physician membership organizations said that if such cuts occurred, physicians would stop seeing Medicare patients and not take any new ones. Medicare, next to Medicaid, was already the lowest insurance payer for physician services. Since physicians are also business people and need to keep their doors open and pay expenses and their employees, they would take only the higher-paying private health insurance patients. At a time when we needed to have more Medicare coverage for our aging population of senior citizens we had created a dynamic in which this care was going to be denied. Therefore, the "SGR freezes" were used to encourage physicians to keep existing Medicare patients and take on new ones, preserving Medicare patients' access to care. Congress has not corrected this formula and has continued to freeze the cuts to physician Medicare payments. This has now led to a nearly $300 billion Medicare debt to the federal government and a pending nearly 30 percent across the board pay cut to physicians for services to Medicare patients until the formula is straightened out.

MANAGED CARE

Costs continued to escalate as new science, technology, and medications skyrocketed, not only in the United States but across the world in the 1970s, 1980s, and 1990s. These health care costs were spiraling out of control and needed to be contained. The health care spend portion of GDP was on its way from approximately 8.9 percent in 1980, to 12 percent in 1990, and 13.6 percent in 1993. This led to entrepreneurial and innovative thinking around how to best manage cost. Organizations sprung into existence in which networks of physicians, hospitals, and other providers were linked together by a managed care system responsible for controlling both financing and costs. This was a very capitalistic, free-market approach and accomplished much of what it set out to do. The cost curve was flattened and the number of people enrolled in managed care organizations increased from 9 to 36 million (11). However, a backlash grew from this process in which patients, physicians, and hospitals lost the personal connection to a caring, trusted physician in favor of a business-like approach to medicine. This left many people disillusioned and staring straight into the eyes of administrators making decisions as opposed to their physicians. Many patients were uprooted from the trusted relationship with their personal primary care doctor and were forced into health maintenance organizations (HMOs) or preferred provider organizations (PPOs). This created great consternation for patient and physician alike. Lawsuits by both physicians and patients were filed against these organizations. America felt that although managed care was a mechanism of controlling cost, it often denied services and lacked much in the humaneness of the interaction. Managed care had forgotten one of the basic tenants of health care: a personal interaction with someone you trust and who cares about you as a person. What was lost was the very critical patient–doctor relationship in which health care is leveraged and made meaningful for patients. What was lost and sacrificed on the altar of the managed care movement was the "profession" of medicine as opposed to the "business" of medicine. Medicine had become more about the cost than about the person, though America and its physicians rejected this premise.

Because of this, major health care reform efforts languished, the status quo flourished, and the medical-industrial complex turned its great economic engine more on wealth generation than health generation. The number of uninsured continued to grow, costs continued to spiral out of control, the lack of access to primary care physicians mounted, creating a wider divide between the haves and the have-nots, especially in health care. This divide widened with our nation's financial crisis and growing national financial debt. Disparities and health care inequities surged and we as a nation continued to kick the health care can down the road for another president and another moment in time.

MEDICARE MODERNIZATION ACT (MMA)

This bill was passed by Congress in 2003 and signed by President George W. Bush into law. It provided the largest overhaul to Medicare since 1965. It created a Medicare prescription drug program that was sorely lacking from the earlier Medicare legislation. Unfortunately, the cost of this program was inaccurately reported when it narrowly passed Congress and its initial price tag of $434 billion now has a 10-year estimate of $1.2 trillion (12). This law also created the very unpopular "donut hole" in Medicare prescription drug coverage. This "donut hole" is a gap in coverage that starts at $2,830 in accumulated prescription medication spending. Patients are then on their own for all prescription costs until $4,550 in expense is reached (13, 14). This is a problem for most senior citizens on Medicare who are living on fixed incomes.

THE VETERANS AFFAIRS, THE DEPARTMENT OF DEFENSE, AND THE INDIAN HEALTH SERVICE

Despite weaknesses in the public and private sector with Medicare,

Medicaid, and private insurance companies, the federal government has created health care systems for veterans, soldiers, sailors, and airmen, and their dependents, and for our Native American populations in the United States, which have been successful.

The VA health care system started in 1930. It has grown from its initial 54 hospitals to its current 171 medical centers, 350 outpatient community clinics, and 126 nursing home units. The VA serves about 8 million enrollees and is budgeted about $100 billion per year (15). The Department of Defense military health system predates the Civil War, and health care benefits to a service member's family (in the form of a single-payer health care system) came about in 1956. The military health system is a $42 billion system that supplies care to 9 million beneficiaries in over 63 military hospitals and over 500 military health clinics (16). The Indian Health Service (IHS) is a $4 billion per year health system serving 2 million Native Americans through 48 hospitals and 230 clinics in 35 states. The IHS was created by the Snyder Act in 1921 and was modified by Congress in 1976 (17). These efforts are pure examples of a government-run national health care system and it has been my direct observation that these government-run systems of care have been outstanding.

These programs have a basic premise that there are no health care bills sent to the patients. All the physicians, hospitals, and personnel are provided and paid for by the federal government. There are minimal differences in physicians' salaries other than those based on years of experience and rank. There are no further incentives for working on quantity or volume or for doing more things to people. These health care systems can also have their problems (e.g., access, waiting times, complexity, lack of primary care, lack of subspecialty care), but they also control costs very well and provide universal high-quality, sustainable care to all of their patients. The federal government created these programs to ensure that these populations were cared for because they can be overlooked by our current health care system. These systems of health care have resulted in high-quality, sustainable care and can be seen as models of care for broadening health care to our nation as a whole.

In conclusion, after reviewing the many events outlined in this chapter, it can be argued that our nation has approached health care and coverage in a very patchwork fashion. On one hand we have reached out to vulnerable and disenfranchised groups. The elderly, the poor, our veterans, our military and their family members, and our Native Americans have been given basic health care through governmental programs such as Medicare, Medicaid, the VA, the Department of Defense health care system, and the Indian Health Service. Over 100 million people are covered by these programs. One-third of Americans are fully covered and cared for by the federal government. It's trying to figure out how best to care for the other two-thirds that presents the majority of the problem. Those with employer-based health insurance or private insurance policies are at least covered, or partially covered, as long as they are employed and can afford it. Those who are not covered (50 million Americans), however, are one heartbeat and one diagnosis away from potential catastrophe and financial ruin.

Table 2 below summarizes the historical events discussed in this chapter along with major issues associated with each one. When cast in this light it becomes very easy to see that as a nation we have progressively narrowed our focus from providing health insurance to everyone to instead selectively focusing on just those who can pay for their own health care. Over the last 65 years, we have selectively decreased the framework of who should be covered by health care. This analysis again raises the question: is health care a basic American right or a money-based privilege? This historic overview frames the question of who ought to pay for what and how should this be funded. As can be seen from this table, our efforts to cover all Americans has shrunk, admittedly with several notable exceptions carved out for selected groups of our population.

Table 2. The Progressive Narrowing of the Intent of Health Care for All Over Time

HISTORICAL EVENT	WHAT WAS THE ISSUE?
National Health Insurance (1945)	Proposed health insurance for all Americans paid for by the federal government and to be funded using taxpayer money obtained from graduated income tax
Private Community Rated Health Insurance (1940–1950s)	Health insurance provided by individual companies available to specific, broad populations of Americans with premiums shared equally by all in the plan independent of age, sickness, etc.
For-Profit Experience Rated Health Insurance (1950s–present)	Health insurance only to selected groups of Americans with costs and qualifications for joining insurance plan dependent on customer's age, preexisting conditions, illnesses, etc.
Medicare and Medicaid (1965-present)	Health insurance paid by the federal government but only for the old, disabled, and/or extremely poor
Competing National Health Plans of the Early 1970s	Ultimately additional health care support for no one
The Late 1970s	Ultimately additional health care support for no one
The Clinton Era (1990s)	Aside from some adjustments to Medicaid and expanded coverage to children (CHIP), added new health care support to no one else
Managed Care	Focused on health care costs first and often put patients' needs second
Medicare Modernization Act	Channeled $1.2 trillion to drug companies
The Veterans Affairs, the DOD, and the Indian Health Service	Created an effective and well-run health care system but was unavailable to anyone who was not a veteran, in the military, or a Native American

Source: Ted Epperly, MD, and Greg Armstrong, PhD

Our country's journey along the path of health care reform has been instructive. As the cost of health care has increased, we have tried to develop mechanisms to provide Americans with protection from those costs, attempted multiple forms of health insurance to meet this need and even passed into law mandated protection for certain populations of Americans to ensure protection from these strangling costs and to ensure they can afford to receive health care. The United States has seen the emergence of employer-based health insurance as a perk to employees to help employers recruit and retain a productive workforce. Health care costs have risen rapidly as an out-of-control expense to employers, employees, individuals, unions, states and our federal government. To this point in time no intervention has had a meaningful and sustainable impact on curbing these rapidly escalating costs while at the same time promising accessible care with high quality outcomes. Those engaged in health care in this country—hospitals, physicians, nurses, health insurance companies, pharmaceutical manufactures, device manufacturers, lawyers, and others—make a lot of money off this system and have actively opposed efforts to help change the health care system that we have created. This, for better or worse, has become our legacy of trying to fix our health care system.

Our nation has been torn by the opposing concepts of wealth versus health and have seen moments of inspired leadership to moments of outright greed. We have seen moments of caring for our fellow man to moments of turning a blind eye to the plight of our fellow man. Our country has seen moments of government intervention and of believing as a nation that health care should be a basic right of all Americans to moments of absolutely rejecting that health care is a basic right to Americans. A patchwork of a health care system has developed that ensures that those with means or in certain patient categories are covered and those without means are on their own in a wildly expensive and fragmented health care system.

Having looked at our history of our health care reform efforts, let's now take a look at what other countries have done with their health care systems for their citizens and what those outcomes have been compared to ours. Are there lessons to be learned from other countries that are instructive in our quest to find the "right" health care system? Is there a "right" health care system? Just what have other countries done?

Chapter 5

HOW DOES OUR HEALTH CARE SYSTEM COMPARE TO OTHER COUNTRIES?

Health care is an effort made to maintain or restore health, usually performed by trained and licensed professionals. Health care can be seen as a system of providing services to people to address acute illness, chronic disease, injury, and to avoid disease, illness, and injury through prevention. The act of providing health care, therefore, is a process. Health, on the other hand, is an outcome. The ideal goal of a health care system should be to generate or restore health to an individual, a community, or to a nation.

All countries participate in health care in one way or another with differing levels of success. This chapter will focus on comparing the United States health care system with other health care systems of the industrialized world. I will analyze each country's strengths, weaknesses, and their challenges. I will then describe our country's health care system and its ability to generate health.

It has become clear to me that there is no one right health care system anywhere in the world. In fact, once you have seen one country's health care system, you have seen only one country's health care system. They are all uniquely different and have come to represent a country's culture, ideology, politics, and its people. If providing health care to a country's people were easy and there was one, best way to do this, we would have similar health care systems in our nations and the problem of how best to provide health care would have been solved long ago. However, the reality has demonstrated that this is not easy and that there is not one perfect way to go about providing health care to a country's people. Tip O'Neil, the former speaker of the House of Representatives, said, "All politics are local." I would say all health care is local as well. Health care must make sense to the people it is there to help and serve or else it is irrelevant.

It is interesting to note that as the United States contemplates a more nationalized health care system, other countries with existing degrees of nationalized health care are moving back toward more privatized, market-driven systems. It reminds me of the old saying that the grass is always greener on the other side of the fence, and underscores the fact that there is not one right or simple way to solve this complex equation. Sorting out the intricacies of cost, access, quality, health care outcomes, patient satisfaction, free choice, while providing social justice to all the people of a country is a daunting undertaking. The answers to health care reform do not lie in extremes. The best health care systems will not blindly follow a total free-market, deregulated, capitalistic model. Nor will they lie at the other extreme in the form of a single-payer, exclusively government-run health care system. The reason for this is that the equation is just too complicated with way too many variables and too many people and special interests to satisfy.

One useful way to classify the world's various health care systems is by examining their sources of payment and their sources of providers. Figure 1 illustrates this. As the figure shows, payment can be either from a single government source; or, in contrast, payment can come from multiple sources such as individual, employer, or government insurance programs, or from out-of-pocket payments from the uninsured. The sources of providers can similarly be broken down into two large categories. The first consists of physicians and other health care providers in independent or private practice arrangements. The second consists of physicians and other providers as government employees.

Figure 1. Health Care Systems of the World

Sources of Payment

	Single Source (Government)	**Multiple Sources** (Individual, Employer, and Government Insurance Programs)
Private or Independent	Canada South Korea Taiwan United States • Medicare • Medicaid • Tricare	Germany France Switzerland Netherlands United States • Employer Insurance • Individual Insurance
Government Employed or Large System Employed	United Kingdom Norway Spain Italy United States • Veterans Affairs (VA) • Department of Defense (DOD) • Indian Health Service (IHS)	United States (Vertically integrated salaried physicians – nongovernmental) • Kaiser Permanente • Group Health • Mayo Clinic System • Cleveland Clinic System • Geisinger Health Plan • Community Health Centers (CHC's)

Sources of Providers

This categorization basically yields four types of health care systems:

1. **Single-Payer/Private Provider**: This model provides an array of independent physicians, hospitals, and health care services. The government acts as the sole source payer but utilizes independent private doctors and hospitals. Countries that use this model through a national health insurance model include Canada, South Korea, and Taiwan. The United States also provides this type of model for how it runs its large federal programs of Medicare, Medicaid, and the military's Tricare program. All of these are single-payer programs that use private or independent physicians, groups, and systems.

2. **Single-Payer/Government Provider**: This model provides health care systems in countries in which the government controls both the source of payment and the system of providers. Countries that use this model of national health care include the United Kingdom, Norway, Spain, and Italy. The United States also uses this type of system in its large federal programs that provide health care in the VA, Department of Defense, and Indian Health Service. All provide a universal health care system where the payment source and employees are paid and work for their nation's government.

3. **Multi-Payer/Private Provider**: This model provides multiple sources of payment through employers, individuals, and government typically through insurance programs. Insurance companies in these countries typically exist to pay bills only. They are middlemen who receive payment from individual clients, employers, or the federal government and then pay for the medical bills that patients incur in the provision of the patient's health care. The source of this money is typically out-of-pocket in an individual's case, through employee deductions or employer payments if the insurance is an employee benefit, or through taxation for a nation's governmental programs. Typically these countries will set the prices that all the insurance companies will pay and that providers can charge. The countries that fall into this general category include Germany, France, Switzerland, Netherlands, and Japan. The United States also uses these types of programs in about 67 percent of all health care transactions. This is the category where most free-market health care occurs.

4. **Multi-Payer/Government (or Large System) Provider**: As can be seen in this figure, no major country other than the United States falls into the fourth category. In general countries that have gone to the trouble of controlling the

physicians and hospitals in the system have also gone to controlling the payment systems through a single-payer nationalized health insurance. The United States, however, also employs this model in large, integrated, nongovernmental health care systems where large corporations own and pay physicians on fixed salaries which approximates this model. Examples of this are seen in large, vertically integrated health care systems such as with Kaiser Permanente based in California, Group Health in the Puget Sound, Mayo Clinic in Minnesota, Florida, and Arizona, the Cleveland Clinic in Ohio, Geisinger Health Plan in Pennsylvania, and the nation's 1,200 Community Health Centers all across the United States.

OUT-OF-POCKET SYSTEM

Another prominent type of health care system that exists in the world could not be depicted in this table. This typically occurs in the rest of the world where countries are not rich enough nor organized enough to provide basic health care for their people. This is the third world where no organized health care systems exist. These countries can only provide health care totally out-of-pocket from individuals or families who pay for these services to physicians or hospitals in their countries on a fee for service basis. This is a total have and have-not free-for-all that sadly encompasses approximately 80 percent of the world's health care systems. In these health care systems the rich or "connected" get health care. Those who are poor or not connected get sick and die. Examples of countries with this type of health care non-system include Cambodia, India, Egypt, and most of Africa, India, China, and South America (1). Sadly, the United States also has 50 million people in this category as well. These are people who don't get health care or wait until they are critically ill and then obtain health care in high-cost places like emergency rooms and hospitals. They typically live sicker and die younger than other people who have other forms of health care.

The other point that I would like to make from the table in Figure 1, and that has been noted by T.R. Reid in his book, *The Healing of America*, is that the United States health care system is represented in all five of the aforementioned models (1). For those over age 65 we provide a single-payer, privatized national health insurance system like Canada. This is called Medicare. For those who are poor and qualify for Medicaid we again provide a single-payer privatized system. We even provide such care through the military's Tricare insurance program for U.S. soldiers and their dependent families who need to receive care in the general public away from their military posts and hospitals.

For those who are veterans and qualify for the VA, active duty military and their families on military posts, and American Indians and Eskimos, we offer them a single-payer, government-run system like the United Kingdom. This is the care model of the Veterans Health Care System, the Military Health Care System, and the Indian Health System. I should point out that this is the health care system that I trained and worked in for 21 years in the United States Army.

The majority (67 percent) of Americans who have some sort of employer-based insurance or individual insurance policy don't fall into the aforementioned groups. They are in the free-market, multi-payer, private-provider market like Germany, France, or Switzerland.

No countries fall completely into the fourth category of multi-payer but government-employed systems. But as discussed above, if you consider large, vertically integrated health care systems where hospitals and physicians are salaried by the health care system as a substitute for government ownership, then the United States can be considered to have such systems as well. They are represented by the health care systems I have mentioned earlier, among others. Another large group that could fit into this category would be the collection of the Community Health Centers (CHCs), which are federally qualified by the United States government but see patients from all payer categories.

The final category, the uninsured, out-of-pocket category is the saddest of all for our nation as well as the rest of the world. For these 50 million patients we offer them a health care system like Cambodia, Burkina Faso, or rural India (1).

It is because of this patchwork of different types of health care in America that we struggle with controlling cost, quality, access, and fairness to all of our citizens. What the other countries have been able to do is focus on one model and make it work. We have multiple models at play with varying degrees of success.

Having said this, let's now take a look at how the health care systems of the world stack up and what are some of the unique characteristics of each of them. Let's start by investigating the cost of health care systems around the world. The United States spends more on health care as a percentage of our gross domestic product (GDP) than every other country on earth (2). In 2004, 15 percent of our GDP was spent on health care. In 2012, this is closer to 18 percent. This compares to 11 percent in the next closest countries of Switzerland and France, and approximately half that much at 8 percent in Spain, the United Kingdom, and Japan. Part of the reason for this is that we have a lot of things to spend money on in our health care system. We have wonderful procedures, imaging technology, medications, physicians, devices, and hospitals to name a few. As a country we have led the way for the rest of the world in health care innovation, health care technology, and health care research. As a result, the expectation of our culture is that getting good care means getting a lot of things done to you. But what also lurks ominously as part of what drives our costs through the roof is our fee-for-service system. The U.S. medical-industrial complex gets paid very well to do things to people. We get paid by volume and paid generously to do things in quantity. In our system, sadly, more leads to more. It's what a capitalistic system rewards.

Figure 2 below demonstrates the average spending on health care per capita. As can be seen in this figure, the United States spends far more than the next closest countries. This spend is approximately

$7,000 per every man, woman, and child as of 2007 (3). As of 2012, this amount has risen to approximately $8,500 per capita.

Figure 2. Average Spending on Health Care Per Capita, 1980–2009

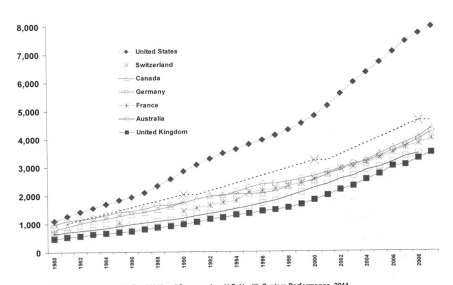

Source: Commonwealth Fund National Scorecard on U.S. Health System Performance, 2011.
Data: OECD Health Data 2011 (database), Version 6/2011.
Modified from: Organisation for Economic Co-operation and Development (2010), "OECD Health Data", OECD Health Statistics (database). doi: 10.1787/data-00350-en (Accessed on 1/26/2012).

Just as Switzerland was next to us in the percent of GDP spent on health care, it also stands to reason that it is the second leading per capita spender at about $4,000 per every man, woman, and child. This compares to about $2,000 per person in New Zealand and the Netherlands. Another item noted in this figure is the precipitous rise in United States' spending over the last 25 years. Unregulated, uncontrolled payment and overutilization of services has led to precipitous spending. This trend, coupled with an aging America and more people with chronic diseases, is creating a fiscal time bomb, a bomb that is ticking.

What portion of the total does each country's public sector

pay for health care for its people? In other words, how much of health financing is seen as a public responsibility? Significantly, the United States is next to the bottom of 30 listed countries at 45.8 percent (4). Public sector spending for health care ranges from a high in Luxembourg of approximately 91 percent to the lowest being that of Mexico at 44.2 percent. The Organization for Economic Cooperation and Development (OECD) has as its average about 73 percent being spent by the public sector on behalf of health care for its people. The OECD is an international organization established in 1961 consisting of 31 countries whose aim is to help governments tackle the economic, social, and governance challenges of a globalized economy. Therefore, even though the United States ranks number one in the world in GDP spending and number one in the world on per capita spending per man, woman, and child, most of those dollars are coming from the private sector through employer-based insurance or from the people themselves and not from the government or public sector. In fact, we have one of the smallest contributions by any country into the health of our country's citizens per capita. This in part is because we do not, as a nation, see health care as being the responsibility of our government to provide to all Americans. Rather, our country sees this as a shared responsibility of employers, individual citizens, and the state and federal government. The problem is that no one is making sure everyone has basic health care. That can be good or bad. If you are healthy or marginally sick, then you can get away with this. However, if you are sick or in rapidly declining health with no health insurance or usual source of care, you are in trouble.

Since much of our nation's health care is paid for by employer or federally sponsored insurance, how do our administrative costs stack up? The United States has roughly a 7.2 percent net health insurance administration cost as a percent of national health expenditures as of 2006, the highest in the industrialized world (5). While the administrative overhead cost of Medicare at 1.5 percent and Medicaid at 5 percent are much lower than those of the for-profit, private health insurance companies (6, 7), private insurance companies have an administrative overhead of around 16.7 percent (8, 9). In other words, United States health insurance companies have higher overhead costs than other countries and even our own Medicare or Medicaid programs. Why? Because private, for-profit health insurance companies spend a lot of time, money, and effort on armies of people whose sole jobs are to collect premiums, pay insurance claims, and deny care to their policyholders. If for-profit health insurance companies can avoid paying health care expenses, then those monies are kept as profit, which helps pay employees and management salaries and sends money to the stockholders of the health insurance company. We therefore have a very unhealthy dynamic in our for-profit health insurance industry. Instead of the money staying in health care, it is siphoned off to profit. The percentage of every dollar that is spent on actually providing medical care is called the "medical loss ratio" by the health insurance industry (telling, don't you think?). In the United States this runs from about 75 percent to 90 percent, which means that only 75 cents to 90 cents of every dollar is spent on actual medical care. Most for-profit health insurance companies keep their medical loss ratios at about 80 percent (10). Therefore, about 20 cents on every dollar is not spent on health care but on administrative overhead, marketing, publications, advertising, denying claims, and denying coverage, again compared to only about 1.5 cents to 5 cents per dollar spent on these activities in the Medicare and Medicaid programs respectively (6, 7). The rest of the industrialized countries spend from about 2 percent to 5 percent of their health care costs on this administration, with the OECD median being 3.4 percent (5). This is another one of the big reasons that health care is so costly in our country.

Let's now shift our focus somewhat and start looking at actual procedural and imaging costs. The United States has roughly 145 coronary bypass procedures per 100,000 people, whereas the OECD median is roughly 61 coronary bypass procedures per 100,000 (11). Do we have more coronary artery disease than other countries? In part yes, but more to the point, this demonstrates that America has a lot of health care services that it offers its people and is not shy about using them. Not only does it offer a lot of procedures, it performs a lot of procedures. Why? Because our system pays, and pays handsomely, for these procedures to be done. These procedures don't even have to be done well. They don't even have to be medically indicated; they just need to be done to be paid for. The payment system fosters things to be done to people and not things to be done well or, better yet, prevented from being done to people in the first place. This in part has helped drive our health care system's overutilization of procedures. So as can be seen, we have a crazy system. The yin and yang is palpable. We have a delivery system that gets paid to do things to people instead of preventing them in the first place. On the other hand, we have a payer system (insurance companies) that tries to deny paying for the procedures and uses loopholes to prevent their payments for these services. Just check your health insurance statement sometime and see if you can make sense of why so little of the costs are paid for and what you owe. And if this is not bad enough, do you think that the health insurance companies pay for prevention? Not on your life. Why? It only stands to reason that they could save money expenditures if they could incentivize prevention and save many procedures from occurring. The rationale is that these savings are too long term. The expense of paying for prevention in the short term does not justify the savings in the long term because most patients will have moved on to another insurance company before the benefits from the cost savings of prevention can be realized by the current insurance company. In fact, most people will have their health insurance plans change from one company to another about every two years. Thus these investment costs in prevention just add to the "medical loss ratio" of the for-profit health insurance companies in the short term, and since the patient will most likely not be with them years from now, why pay for this now? Let's just kick that can down the road.

So what about our country's use of imaging services? The United States has more CT scanners than any other country at approximately 32 CT scanners per million people (12). The United States has 27 MRI scanners per million people. The number of MRI scanners in the United States is only exceeded by Japan. By the way, the OECD median for number of MRI scanners in 30 industrialized countries is 7.7 per million people. This compares to the previously mentioned 27 per million in the United States (12). This is nearly four times more than the OECD average. This again underscores that America loves our technology and tends to do what it gets paid to do, and that is to do procedures and imaging. When technology is perceived in our country as the way to make diagnoses and to cure problems, then everyone expects to have these done. It is our country's health care culture. In addition, liability concerns and fears of being sued drive a tendency to require that procedures be done and done and done again. Now, of course having all these MRI units and CT scanners allows our citizens to be able to get these services fairly easily without waiting lines. Therefore, access, convenience, and ease of utilization are better in the United States than elsewhere in the world for those who have health insurance or the means to pay. However, the question must be asked, are all these images necessary? This somewhat mindless overuse of technology is exactly what can lead to higher dollars per capita being spent on health care.

The other major issue of course is the cost of these scans. For instance, the cost of an MRI scan of the brain in the United States is $1,000 to $1,400. In Japan the cost of that same MRI is $105 (13). America by contrast to the other countries of the world is over-imaged, over-procedured, over-priced, and generally overdone when it comes to health care. It is this variation in utilization and gaps of care that is part of our crazy system. And what about the health risks of all of this ionizing radiation? Are we doing more harm than good? Not only this, but what about the questionable findings seen on these

MRIs and CT scans that are normal variations or are not harmful at all that then result in more studies, tests, and procedures? Doing more things to people can be harmful, even dangerous. More can lead to more, and more can be toxic to people's health. As a country we must all become more aware and educated on when enough is enough and when to stop.

So with all these procedures getting done to Americans, how is our health doing? What do we get for the privilege of being over-imaged and over-operated on? Figure 3 below shows the World Health Organization (WHO) health care rankings for the top 55 nations. As can be seen, despite all of our spending as a country per individual on CT scanners, MRI scanners, and coronary by-pass procedures and everything else, this buys us a rank of number 37 in the world (14). Behind the countries of Colombia, Cyprus, Saudi Arabia, United Arab Emirates, Morocco, Dominica, and Costa Rica.

Figure 3. World Health Organization Health System Performance in All Member States

Rank	Member State	Rank	Member State	Rank	Member State	Rank	Member State	Rank	Member State
1	France	11	Norway	21	Belgium	31	Finland	41	New Zealand
2	Italy	12	Portugal	22	Colombia	32	Australia	42	Bahrain
3	San Marino	13	Monaco	23	Sweden	33	Chile	43	Croatia
4	Andorra	14	Greece	24	Cyprus	34	Denmark	44	Qatar
5	Malta	15	Iceland	25	Germany	35	Dominica	45	Kuwait
6	Singapore	16	Luxembourg	26	Saudi Arabia	36	Costa Rica	46	Barbados
7	Spain	17	Netherlands	27	United Arab Emirates	37	United States of America	47	Thailand
8	Oman	18	United Kingdom	28	Israel	38	Slovenia	48	Czech Republic
9	Austria	19	Ireland	29	Morocco	39	Cuba	49	Malaysia
10	Japan	20	Switzerland	30	Canada	40	Brunei Darussalam	50	Poland

Source: WHO. The World Health Report 2000. *Health Systems: Improving Performance.* 2000; 209.

How are such rankings determined? They come from evaluating metrics such as life span and infant mortality. They include comparisons of health care system efficiency, equity, responsiveness, and fairness. Not everyone in our country gets uniform care, which leads to wide disparities in quality, access, and health care outcomes. So, for example, when it comes to having a fair, just, and equitable system, the United States ranks 54th in the world (15), even worse than our 37th place overall average ranking.

So what about life expectancy, arguably the gold standard for a health care system? The length and quality of one's life is important to people. Of the 11 industrialized countries, the United States ranks 11th out of 11 (16). The OECD median is approximately two years more of extended life span for men and for women when compared to the United States. In other words, for the privilege of all of our testing, all of our technology, and the exorbitant amounts of money we pay as a health care system, we live two years less than the other industrialized nations.

Another useful indicator is "avoidable mortality," which looks at how well a country does at curing curable diseases (17). The Commonwealth Fund in 2008 ranked the United States 19th out of 19 of the wealthy countries (18). Another Commonwealth Fund study of nine developed countries showed that Americans with diabetes, kidney transplants, major surgery, and death rates due to surgical or medical mishaps were the worst of the nine (17, 19). For asthma, we ranked seventh of nine countries. In another category of "health life expectancy at age 60," as determined by the Commonwealth Fund in a 2006 survey, the United States came in tied for 23rd place of 23 countries (17, 20). The lesson learned from all of this is that having all the technology, hardware, imaging, hospitals, and doctors in the world is not translating into prolonged life expectancy or better health outcomes. It is not translating into better health. When a country like ours focuses on disease, treatment, procedures, and imaging and on payment for these things instead of on meticulous chronic disease management, good nutrition, exercise, weight loss, smoking cessation, decreasing alcohol use, seat belt utilization, and disease prevention, our reward is poorer health. More medicine, more procedures, and more imaging can be toxic to people. Not only are they more expensive and costly, they can also injure and kill people through medical error, and can make our collective lives shorter.

I know I have hammered hard on this point, but as a family physician, who focuses on my patients' and community's health, there is one more study I want to share. If you compare the six countries of Australia, Canada, Germany, New Zealand, the United Kingdom, and the United States relative to each other and in quality of care, access, efficiency, equity, health expenditures per capita, and its people living long, healthy, and productive lives, the United States ranks sixth of these six countries (21). We struggle collectively with quality, coordination, access, efficiency, equity, and length of our lives. And for the privilege of all of that, we also pay the most. In fact, we pay double to triple these other countries' amounts. So we have room for health care system improvements around cost, access, quality, and almost every other parameter when compared with the rest of our brothers and sisters in the world. This is not because other countries have better innovations or brighter people. They simply have better health care *systems* than we do. They integrate and coordinate. We fragment and partialize. Where they work as teams, we work as individuals. They do not have any better individuals. They have better teams and systems. They have better insurance systems. They are more efficient than we are.

Now, in making comparisons across the world, it is important to point out that there are unique differences among countries even as we all engage in caring for our citizens. For many of the disease conditions, such as cancer, heart failure, pneumonia, and AIDS, we have some of the best health care in the world (22). There is no doubt that we have the most robust research infrastructure, technologic and pharmaceutical innovation, and Nobel Prize winners than anywhere else in the world. However, all of this comes at a cost and the ability to pay for it. We see large disparities in health care: people with means can obtain the fruits of what the health care system has to offer, whereas those without the means cannot. That leads to large segments of the population having uneven care, which is part of the problem in why our quality outcomes do not rank as well.

What the European Union and other OECD nations have been able to do in the industrialized world is norm around the concept of *solidarity* in the belief that health care is a basic right of all the citizens of its country. These nations have created a health care system within their countries so that *all* people have basic health care coverage and access. Where costs are subsidized and health versus disease is promoted. In contrast, what we have struggled with in our country is the ability to norm around this basic concept of solidarity of ensuring that everyone has access to basic health care. This is what leads to disparities in health care and large gaps in quality outcomes over the greater population of the United States. If every citizen cannot obtain basic health care, then large holes in quality are going to exist, and they do. In response, the United States focuses more on disease than health and has a broadly discrepant have and have-not health system. While other countries have solid, intact health care systems the United States has a health care system that looks like Swiss cheese.

Now, let's take a look at some of the countries ranked by the World Health Organization in its top 20. These are larger countries with democracies similar to our own. We will look at not only their strengths but also their weaknesses.

FRANCE

France has been considered by the World Health Organization as having the best health care system in the world (14, 23). Its quality outcomes are high and its life expectancy is at the top. Its system provides universal coverage with 99 percent of its people covered by national health insurance (24). This provides a basic package of health care, which includes inpatient and outpatient care, physician and specialist services, home care service, diagnostic testing, and prescription medications. The French people have a health card that allows them health care access anywhere in France. Not only does this card allow them to receive care, but it is encrypted with the person's demographic and medical information so all of this can be easily uploaded at the point of care. Similarly, once the medical visit is over, the new information can be uploaded onto this card. This is truly medical care in the Information Age.

The French government runs somewhat like a utility in setting premiums, benefits, and provider reimbursement rates. However, like many other countries, it struggles with cost control, with its health care costs as a percentage of GDP being third in the world at approximately 11 percent and its per capita spending being fourth in the world at about $3,200 per person (2, 3). Co-pays are levied at approximately 10 percent to 40 percent of the cost to help put some skin in the game from the French people to help control utilization. Having said this, only 13 percent of their health care costs are out-of-pocket. The French people pay approximately 18.8 percent of their income for health insurance. Additionally, there are dedicated taxes on alcohol, tobacco, and pharmaceutical company revenues. The French have considered moving towards a system of managed care that tries to provide a preferred provider and a pathway of care for a particular problem. If one goes outside that pathway, then additional charges can occur. This has not gone over well with the French citizens because choice has become an important principle to them in their health care system. The French are using a bit of a hybrid system where not only do they have their nationalized health insurance with 99 percent of the people being covered, but 92 percent of their people have private insurance as well. This system is unique to France, but it works well for the French people and they are very happy with their health care system. Controlling costs and improving efficiencies are their biggest challenges.

ITALY

The Italian health care system is ranked number two in the world by the World Health Organization and spends approximately 9 percent of its GDP on health care (2). The Italian system has its federal government provide basic rules and regulations that are then implemented in a decentralized fashion by local health authorities spread across the nation. The financing of the Italian system comes from payroll taxes and general revenues as well as federal and regional general taxation. This provides basic health care coverage to all the Italian citizens. This includes primary care and inpatient care that are free. Co-payments are charged, however, for such services as specialists, diagnostic procedures, and prescription drugs. Approximately 10 percent of Italians have additional private health insurance. An additional 35 percent pay out-of-pocket for private health services when deemed needed (25). Unfortunately, spiraling costs and waiting lines do plague the Italian health care system as this country continues to determine how to most effectively deliver health care to its people.

SPAIN

The Spanish health care system ranks seventh in the world and spends approximately 8 percent of its GDP on health care (2). It provides nationalized health insurance to all of its citizens per the Spanish Constitution, yielding 98.7 percent of its people with coverage. It works in a highly decentralized fashion, with 17 Spanish regions receiving block grants to be spent as they see fit for the health care of their people (26). Primary care physicians and specialists are assigned to the citizenry based on geographic location. Spain lacks enough primary care physicians as well as nurses and is in crisis similarly to the United States in this regard. This leads to long wait times for access to health care. This is compounded by long wait times to see specialists as well. Because of this, there is a movement towards private insurance, with about 12 percent of the Spanish population purchasing private insurance and 24 percent of Spaniards paying out-of-pocket expenses to obtain additional care (26). Despite this challenge, the Spanish people are satisfied with their health care, ranking second of the European Union countries.

JAPAN

Japan's health care system ranks 10th in the world according to the World Health Organization and spends roughly 8 percent of its GDP on health care (2). The Japanese system provides universal health insurance to all of its citizenry through compulsory employment-based insurance. This amounts to about an 8.5 percent payroll tax that is split roughly 50/50 between the employer and the employee. The Japanese system runs on a fee-for-service system and is a high-volume system, with many people being churned through in very rapid times by its physicians. The Japanese people see their physicians on average of 14 times per year, which is the largest number of visits on average per person than anywhere else in the world (27). By comparison, the average number of visits per person in the United States is three to four visits per year. Only about 1 percent of the Japanese health care system's spending is by additional private insurance and about 17 percent is by out-of-pocket spending. Of interest, there is no difference between inpatient and outpatient fees, which has tended to drive the system to do much more in the outpatient versus the inpatient sector (28). The Japanese people have a strong aversion to invasive procedures, so surgical fees and invasive radiologic fees are lower proportionally to other fees. The Japanese system is driven by a lot of noninvasive technology, and Japan leads the world with the number of MRI scanners at 40 per million people (12). Since Japan's population is rapidly aging, similar to the United States, Japan faces a looming health care crisis. The biggest challenges for the Japanese health care system are overutilization of health care and the having the most hospitals per person in the world. This has led to a mal-distribution of care among the types of physicians Japan needs and the geographic distribution with the rural areas being undersupplied (29).

NORWAY

The health care system in Norway ranks 11th in the world by the World Health Organization and spends about 9.5 percent of its GDP on health care (2). It is a single-payer, tax-funded, universal health care system, in which all the citizens of Norway and anyone else living or working there is covered. The benefits include primary care, inpatient and outpatient care, diagnostic services, maternity services, specialist care, preventive medicine, prescription medications, and end-of-life care. There are no charges for care at the public hospitals and there are provisions for sick pay and disability benefits. Primary care physicians are assigned by municipal local authorities, whereas specialist care is assigned and governed by four regional health care authorities (30). The Norwegian government sets an annual budget and fixed salaries are paid to the primary care physicians. Specialists receive both an annual grant and fee-for-service payment. That fee-for-service payment is what has helped as an incentive to decrease wait lines. To ensure a robust primary care workforce the primary care physicians are paid more than any other type of physician, which provides excellent primary care and balanced workforce development. The people of Norway are very satisfied with their health care system, but as with all health care systems in the world, costs are continually monitored as are waiting lines and access to health care.

NETHERLANDS

The Netherlands rank 17th in the World Health Organization rankings and spend approximately 9 percent of its GDP on health care (2). In 2006 the Netherlands put in place a new health care system similar to managed competition, like Switzerland. Under this model, all Dutch citizens must purchase a private health insurance plan from a multitude of private insurance companies. These plans are purchased by each citizen, with the government of Netherlands setting the premiums in a range that can be competed for by the private insurance companies. This is a mandate that has resulted in 98.5 percent of the population being insured. The basic package of benefits includes primary and specialist care, hospital stays, maternity and prenatal care, dental care, some medications, and travel expenses. About 90 percent of the Dutch citizens also purchase supplemental insurance in case they need additional services (31). The payment for this plan is about 50 percent from employers and 50 percent from employees. Subsidies are allowed for the poor on a sliding fee scale. Physicians negotiate with insurance companies for payment, which is also based on quality incentives and performance metrics. This has led to a bit of a free-market competition system in their country, and since the system is only about six years old, it will need to be watched. The biggest challenge of this young health care system in the Netherlands is controlling costs (32).

THE UNITED KINGDOM

The United Kingdom (U.K.) ranks 18th in the world according to WHO health care rankings. It spends approximately 8 percent of its GDP on health care (2). Its average life expectancy for males and females is about a year longer than for American men and two years longer for women (16). It spends about $2,400 per capita on health care in its country (3). The national health service of the U.K. is the prototypical single-payer universal health care system. It is a true "socialized health care system." But as British Health Minister John Reid has said, "We cover everybody, but we don't cover everything." (33) It is highly centralized and funded through general tax revenues with no direct charges to patients. Most of its physicians and nurses are government employees. Basic benefits include primary and specialty care, hospitalizations, diagnostic testing, basic medications, and maternity care. The government of Great Britain struggles with controlling costs and waiting lines as it tries to balance supply and demand while providing quality health care to its people (33). About 10 percent of its citizens have private health insurance, which affords them a broader array of coverage and avoidance of the waiting lines. Despite growing tensions with the health care system in the United Kingdom, the citizens there are extremely proud of it and do not want it to change. The biggest challenges are the appropriate utilization of care and controlling costs (34).

SWITZERLAND

Switzerland's health care system ranks 20th in the world and spends approximately 11.5 percent of its GDP on health care. In this regard, it's second only to the United States in its health care spending but still well ahead of the United States' 17 percent GDP spending on health care (2). The Swiss health care system is also the closest to the United States' system, using a managed competition model where the provision of health care and health insurance resides in the private sector. This has created a highly regulated marketplace from which health care is provided. By Swiss law there is an individual mandate and all Swiss citizens must have health insurance. That results in 99.5 percent of their citizenry having health insurance (35). This insurance is bought from multiple competing insurance companies by individuals. Employers have minimal roles in contributing to the purchase of health insurance. The basic benefits package is fairly robust and includes inpatient and outpatient care, diagnostic testing and prescription drugs, and care for the physically/mentally disabled to include nursing home care. The insurance companies use community rating, meaning that similar costs and benefits are given to all. There is, however, a 20 percent reduction for people who do not smoke. In this Swiss system, approximately 17 percent of total health spending is paid by the government and about 32 percent is paid out-of-pocket (36). The insurance companies compete on their deductibles and co-pays since their other prices are fixed. Subsidies are provided by the Swiss government so that no individual pays more than about 10 percent of their income on insurance. Approximately one-third of the Swiss citizens receive some form of subsidy. Approximately 40 percent of the Swiss citizens also have supplemental insurance, which provides additional services (29). The Swiss style of health care is highly technologic-driven like it is in the United States, which drives up its GDP spending and its spending per capita to roughly $4,100 per Swiss citizen (3). This is still much cheaper than the $8,500 spent in the

U.S. per capita. Life expectancy in Switzerland is about four years longer for men and women than it is in the United States (16). The biggest challenge for the Swiss health care system is controlling cost. It is the most expensive health care system in Europe and second only to the U.S. in the world (37).

GERMANY

Germany ranks 25th in the world according to the WHO health care ranking and has a GDP spending of approximately 11 percent (2). The German people live two years longer on average for men and women than their United States counterparts (16). The German system is a national health insurance system that has been in place since the time of Otto von Bismarck in 1883. This provides health care for everyone with an opt-out function for those who want private insurance. Approximately 90 percent of the German citizens are in its nationalized insurance plan, almost 100 percent of its citizens have some form of insurance, and 9 percent have an additional supplemental insurance (38). The German system pays approximately 75 percent of health care spending in the country with approximately 13 percent being out-of-pocket, which is almost identical to the United States (36). The funds for the German health care system is a payroll tax split approximately equally between employer and employee, which amounts to about 15 percent of the wages. Benefits for the program are extensive and cover primary and specialty care physicians, clinic and hospital care, acute and chronic care, diagnostic testing, preventive care, prescription drugs, and some dental care (38). Cost and prices are escalating in Germany and they are trying to control these by limiting benefits. Germans do not use as much of a technology-driven system as the Swiss or the Americans. The largest challenges looming for the German health care system are similar to the United States: a large and growing aged population, high costs, and high rate of specialist visits (39).

CANADA

The Canadian health care system ranks 30th in the world according to WHO health care ranking and spends approximately 9 percent of its GDP on health care (2). This results in about $3,500 being spent per capita per year in Canada and gives life expectancy of about two and half years longer than the United States citizen (3, 16). The Canadian system is a national health system that is financed jointly by the Canadian government and its provinces. The implementation of the health care is decentralized to Canada's 10 provinces and two territories. The governmental financing comes from general tax revenue that's distributed as a block grant to each of the provinces and territories and constitutes about 16 percent of the total spending in those areas. The additional spending comes from the provinces and territories by having taxes that are personal and corporate, as well as sales taxes and lottery proceeds. Several of the provinces also have premiums. All the provinces and territories provide a basic benefit package that includes primary care physicians, specialists, hospitals, and some degree of dental care. There is some variation, however, across provinces in regards to routine dental care, physical therapy, and prescription drugs. Reimbursement to physicians is set by each province and is a fee-for-service system. There are private insurance companies that are increasing, and these are employer-purchased. Controlling costs have been well done by the Canadian government and have kept this relatively flat at about 9 percent of the GDP; however, waiting times are a problem in Canada (40). The longest waits occur for hip and knee replacements as well as cataract surgery. Some would say since these are elective surgeries they are less urgent and can certainly wait. There is less technology with CT and MRI scanners in Canada than there is in the United States and there are fewer procedures performed (11, 12). Although Canadians know their health care system is not perfect and there are problems with their wait times, amongst others, they clearly look south across the border and realize they have a better overall health care system.

UNITED STATES

As discussed earlier in this chapter, our health care system in the United States is a hodgepodge of multiple systems. In fact, it is a health care non-system that struggles with accountability. It struggles with integration and coordination of care. It is the most expensive health care system in the world and is literally collapsing under its own weight of health care costs. Despite the exorbitant expense of health care at $2.6 trillion per year, we struggle with quality. The United States system ranks 37th in the world according to the World Health Organization and spends 17 percent of its GDP on health care and about $8,500 annually per capita on health care expenses (2, 3, 14). The United States health care system is a managed competition model where employer health insurance coverage accounts for 52 percent, public health insurance in the form of Medicare, Medicaid, and SCHIP accounts for 28 percent, individual health insurance coverage for about 5 percent, and there are approximately 15 percent uninsured (41). Within the public sector's 28 percent, Medicaid represents 14 percent (50 percent), Medicare 12.4 percent (45 percent), and the combination of Indian Health Service and State Children's Health Insurance Program (SCHIP) representing 1 to 2 percent each (41). The amounts of health care expenditures for military and Veterans Affairs (VA) programs are not included in these numbers. The United States system provides some type of health insurance coverage for about 85 percent of its citizens, but the remaining 50 million Americans (16 percent) were without health insurance in 2009.

This system of care is based on a fee-for-service model that focuses on disease treatment, procedures, and imaging and has not focused well on the social determinates of health, disease prevention, and health promotion. It is a highly unstable system with rapid cost growth, premium insurance increases, and overutilization of services. Life expectancy is two years less for men and women than other OECD nations (16).

THE COUNTRIES AND PEOPLE OF "RICHLAND" AND "POORLAND"

Since the United States is such a quilt-work of health care systems all mixed into one, I would like to create a thought experiment with our country subdivided into two different imaginary countries. These two countries would be "Richland" for the wealthiest people in our country and "Poorland" for the poorest people in the United States. This thought experiment will help frame the have and have-not system of health care we have in the United States. Figure 4 compares and contrasts some of the health care expenditures, procedures, and outcomes of these two imaginary countries within the United States.

Figure 4. A Comparison of "Richland," "Poorland," and the United States

	"Richland"	"Poorland"	United States
Education Level	16+	10	13.3
Average Income	$100,000+	$20,000	$40,566
Percent with Health Insurance	99%	20%	85%
Total Expenditures on Health as Percent of GDP	20%	3%	16%
Dollars Spent on Health Per Year	$10,000	$1,500	$7,500
Out-of-Pocket Health Care Spending Per Capita	$600	$1,300	$857
Number of MRI Units Per Million People	45	1	27
Number of CT Units Per Million People	45	3	33
Coronary Artery Bypass Procedures (CABP) Per 100,000	300	30	145

	"Richland"	"Poorland"	United States
WHO Performance – Overall Health Care Rankings	5	112	37
Life Expectancy at Birth – Males	80	64	75.2
Life Expectancy at Birth – Females	90	74	80.4
Primary Care Physicians Per 100,000	40	10	30
Subspecialist Physicians Per 100,000	100	20	70

"Richland" is a thriving country of professionals and white-collar jobs where people are very well educated, with over 16 years of formal education and earn incomes in excess of $100,000 year. Ninety-nine percent of its citizens have excellent insurance policies.

"Poorland" is a struggling country where most people are laborers and in blue-collar jobs or, worse yet, have no jobs. They are not well educated and they need to get into the job market to earn a living and to start making money. Therefore, they average about 10 years of formal education and average yearly salaries of approximately $20,000 per year.

The people of Richland spend much more on health care as a part of their nation's gross domestic product than the people of Poorland. This is because they have more technology and Cadillac insurance plans that cover all types of procedures and imaging. Because of this, the people of Richland tend to overutilize the health care system. They get more things covered and paid for than those in Poorland who either have no insurance at all or have very skimpy insurance policies in which they are underinsured and have little access to procedures and imaging. This overutilization leads to more medicine, more procedures, more consultations, more of everything in Richland compared to Poorland. This has a direct impact in the amount of money spent per individual in these two countries per year and the resulting spend of the nation as a whole in its gross domestic product (GDP). As noted in Figure 4, this leads to $10,000 spent on Richland's health care per year and only $1,500 spent by Poorland's citizens. This is also reflected in the effect on health care spending by these two nations as a whole with Richland spending 20 percent of its GDP on health care and Poorland spending 3 percent. In comparison, it can be seen that the real country of the United States spends $8,500 on every man, woman, and child per year, which represents 17 percent of our GDP. As noted earlier in this chapter and throughout this book, this is by far the most outlay for any country in the world. The country of Richland would be even higher than the United States. Part of the reason for this is that the cultural expectation of Richland is that you can get any type of medical care whenever you want it. "More medicine must be better medicine" is what the citizens of Richland have come to expect. Conversely, the people of Poorland have come to expect just the opposite. They have come to expect very little health care unless you can pay for it or are part of Poorland's military or privileged elected leaders. In fact, most of Poorland citizens avoid and do not seek out health care.

This leads to a very distorted out-of-pocket spending in these two countries as well. Since Poorland has very little health insurance and most people who do have health insurance are underinsured, this leads to large out-of-pocket expenditures of $1,300 per year. This compares to only $600 for the better-insured people of Richland. The people of Poorland are paying 87 percent ($1,300-$1,500) of all their health care costs out-of-pocket. And those costs are the full costs and not the discounted costs that the people of Richland pay because their insurance companies have negotiated lower rates with hospitals and physicians. The people of Richland pay only 6 percent of their health care costs per year out-of-pocket ($600 of the $10,000 spent on health care per year) so they don't understand why more people in Poorland don't get better health care.

These differences in income between Richland and Poorland and the wealth of the two nations as a whole leads to an incredible difference in regards to what medical things get done in these two countries. Remember one of the important themes I mentioned earlier in the book is that what gets paid for gets done. The other major theme is that all you need to do to figure out much about health care in the United States is to follow the flow of money.

Richland, therefore, has an exorbitant amount of MRI and CT scanners to image the body. Why? Because they can afford them and the people of Richland expect to have MRIs or CT scans whenever they think they need them. Insurance is purchased that pays for these scans and they pay well for them to be done.

Poorland has very few of these MRI and CT scanners. In fact, 45 times less MRI scanners (45 to 1 per million people) and 15 times less CT scanners (45 to 3 per million people). The reason that Poorland has a bit better ratio of CT scanners than MRI scanners when compared to Richland is because the CT scanners are less expensive and older technology. In fact, Poorland purchased many of these older CT scanners from Richland as Richland upgraded to latest and greatest generation of the new MRI and CT scanners.

The differences in these two neighboring countries can also be seen in what types of procedures get done and how easy it is to get them done. The number of coronary artery bypass grafts, or CABGs (pronounced as "cabbages"), is over 10 times greater in Richland than Poorland (300 to 30). Not because the people of "Richland" have more heart disease requiring these operations, but because there is a better system in place to pay for them. Therefore, there are more heart surgeons, more cardiologists, more heart catheterization labs, more heart stints placed, more operating rooms to do open heart procedures like coronary artery bypass grafts in Richland. Poorland, conversely, doesn't have the resources to pay for these procedures or the infrastructure of specialists to support them.

Because of all of these things, the overall world health care rankings and health care outcomes as measured by the World Health Organization for these two countries are markedly different, as one could predict. In Richland the WHO performance for health care outcomes places them fifth in the world. Poorland weighs in at 112th in the world. The real country of the United States weighs in at number 37, in part because of its mixtures of the countries of Richland and Poorland.

For these same reasons, the life expectancy of males and females in Richland exceed those in Poorland by 16 years for men and woman. The reason for this is that the people of Richland have better access to primary care physicians because of their health insurance. Having more scanners and procedures such as CABGs in Richland is not the bottom line in having better health care outcomes than Poorland. It is because the people of Richland have better integrated and coordinated care than Poorland and less fragmentation of care. Therefore, more prevention and wellness medicine and behavior changes such as smoking cessation, obesity prevention, exercise promotion, immunizations, nutrition counseling, substance abuse counseling, and proactive mental health care are provided in Richland than in Poorland. This focus on keeping people well versus just treating them when they are sick goes a long way to improving health care outcomes.

Richland has a greater number of primary care physicians than does Poorland and this helps with prevention and wellness. In fact, the fourfold increase in primary care physicians between the two explains better and more timely access into the health care system. Richland also has more subspecialty physicians as could be predicted by the wealth of the country and what gets paid for in the country. Since surgeries, procedures, and imaging are well paid for, these subspecialty doctors flourish. In Poorland these subspecialty physicians are not well paid and hence there are less of them, which makes both integrated primary care and timely subspecialty care hard to come by. In fact, many of the primary care physicians and subspecialty care physicians leave Poorland and move to Richland as their incomes can be significantly increased, which only worsens the access to primary care and the provision of quality care across the entire country of Poorland.

As can be seen from our thought experiment, we have two incredibly different health care systems based on the ability to have meaningful health insurance and access to a primary care physician for a usual source of health care. We also have wildly divergent health care systems based on the wealth of the nation and what it has decided as a country to value.

Although this particular diagram is totally fictitious, it makes the point that we have a disparate quality of care in the United States based on socioeconomics, what part of town, state, or county you live in, education level, ability to access care, whether you have health insurance or not, and income. Just as in America now, the people of Poorland live sicker and die younger than those in Richland.

WHAT DOES THIS MEAN TO RICHARD AND PAUL?

Let's take this thought experiment one step further and bring it down from a national level to an individual level. From Richland we will have a 58-year-old man named Richard. From Poorland we will have a 58-year-old man named Paul. Both Richard and Paul are hard-working men who care deeply about their communities and their families. They both are happily married with two children each. Richard works as a bank vice president with a great health insurance plan he gets through his bank. Paul works in a small grocery store where his employer cannot afford health insurance for his three employees. Richard's wife does not need to work outside of the home. Paul's wife does and she works as a motel maid in which there is also no health insurance. Both Richard and Paul developed hypertension in their 30s. Richard knew this and was on medication. Paul did not know this and was not put on any medication.

Two months ago, each of these men started to experience chest pain while working. Richard decided to see his primary care physician who became immediately concerned with the squeezing quality of the chest pain and his associated shortness of breath. His physician placed him on nitroglycerin tablets to put under his tongue if this pain returned, told him to not exercise or exert himself, and set him up for an exercise treadmill in his office two days later.

Paul, on the other hand, was concerned with his squeezing chest pain and shortness of breath, but since he had no health insurance or primary care physician decided to give this pain some time, trying not to walk as much and take it a little easier.

Richard, two days later, when tested on the exercise treadmill by his primary care physician was markedly positive for exercise-induced chest pain (angina) and had positive electrocardiogram changes consistent with coronary artery disease. His physician set him up immediately with a referral to a cardiologist the next day.

Paul conversely noted his chest pain now started to develop when at rest, but because it only lasted two to three minutes, he decided to slow down his activity level a little bit more.

Richard was seen by the cardiologist the next day and was set up for a heart catheterization the day after that. During the heart catheterization he was noted to have a major obstruction of his left main coronary artery. This obstruction was 90 percent of the artery's internal diameter. The cardiologist was unable to place a coronary artery stent that would prop open the coronary artery and he was told by the cardiologist that he needed immediate referral to a cardiac surgeon for an urgent coronary artery bypass graft (CABG).

Paul was now having one to two episodes of his chest pain per day, both with walking and at rest. He decided not to tell his wife or employer since they "had problems of their own" and stick it out a bit longer because he really didn't have any doctor to go and believed that this wasn't a problem to go to the emergency room for. Especially since that visit would cost him over $1,000 for what they would surely tell him was "indigestion."

Richard underwent successful coronary artery bypass grafting and was told by all three of his physicians (his primary care physician, his cardiologist, and his heart surgeon) that he had "dodged a bullet" in having this diseased coronary artery alert him to his heart disease. They told him that this particular blockage is called a "widow maker" because of its propensity to suddenly cause cardiac arrhythmias, heart attack, and death. He was thankful for his good luck, excellent team of physicians, and his health insurance.

Paul, however, did not seek nor receive this care since he could not afford it. The same day Richard had his coronary artery bypass graft performed, Paul had a massive heart attack from the exact same occlusion in his coronary artery. He developed excruciating chest pain, nausea, vomiting, shortness of breath, and pain not only in his chest but also into his left shoulder and arm. His wife called 911 and he was taken to his local hospital where they confirmed his heart attack. His local hospital could not perform his catheterization or his potential surgery, so Paul was air transported from Poorland to a hospital in Richland where they could offer state-of-the-art heart care. In fact, it was the same hospital where Richard was. The cardiologist on call performed a catheterization and confirmed the left main coronary artery obstruction of 98 percent but could not easily place a stent, so he went to urgent coronary artery bypass surgery. In fact, the same cardiologist and heart surgeon who cared for Richard cared for Paul. After the surgery in the surgical intensive care unit, both said to him that your particular blockage is called a "widow-maker" and it's too bad that you didn't know about your hypertension and angina earlier and that you were not seen and treated before you had your massive heart attack.

Richard left the hospital seven days later with a new lease on life.

Paul went into massive heart failure from his heart attack and weakened heart muscle, and died on the seventh postoperative day.

Richard's total out-of-pocket expense was $2,100 of the $65,000 that his primary care visit, cardiologist visit, cardiac catheterization, heart surgery, and hospitalization cost.

Paul's bill to his widow was $95,000 for his transport by ambulance, ER visit, air evacuation by helicopter from Poorland to Richland hospital, the cardiologist, the cardiac catheterization, the heart surgery, and the hospital and intensive care unit (ICU) time.

Richard's wife regained her husband. Paul's wife lost her husband and gained a $95,000 bill that would drive her to declare bankruptcy.

These two thought experiments of Richland and Poorland were intended to help explain the have and have-not nature of our United States health care system in a more graphic way. As can be seen at both a national and an individual level, how one's health care system is constructed can have a profound influence on both an individual citizen and the nation's health outcomes as a whole. These are important issues and fundamental to the fabric of health care, not only in our country but all of the countries of the world.

CONCLUSIONS

So what can we learn from the world's health care systems? In his book *The Health of America, A Global Quest for Better, Cheaper, and Fairer Health Care*, T.R. Reid speaks to three universal laws of health care systems as articulated by the American economist Tsung-Mei Cheng:

1. No matter how good a country's health care is, people will complain about it.

2. No matter how much money is spent on health care, doctors and hospitals will argue that it is not enough.

3. The last reform tried always failed. (42)

These three simple statements ring true to me, and there are other important conclusions that can be drawn from the studies of other countries' health care systems:

- If you have seen one country's health care system, you have seen one country's health care system. There is much uniqueness in systems occurring across our planet, primarily driven by each country's culture, political system, and values.

- There is no perfect health care system anywhere in the world, or we would all copy it. Clearly the United States is not the world's best example, but neither are those of other countries.

Each country is struggling to get the right balance of cost control, access, and quality.

- Experimentation on health care systems will continue as long as people live on this earth. Countries will constantly tweak and innovate to better meet the needs their people, as they should. Technology and information management are constantly changing.

- Since the grass is greener on the other side of the fence, people will continue to look at other countries' health care systems to try to find elusive answers (43). These models may or may not be good for a particular country but can foster innovative thinking.

- Just having insurance for a country's people does not equal health care. Unless the delivery system by physicians, hospitals, and other health care professionals is in place, it will only lead to frustration and waiting lines. Remember the analogy that giving bus passes to everyone in a city with only two buses does not equal transportation? Similarly, giving everyone health care coverage with the wrong types of providers for them to see does not equal health care, let alone health.

- Much of the marked increase in cost of health care is driven by technology and the explosion of scientific research. Countries that use more technology in their health care systems will have problems controlling cost.

- Nationalized health care systems with universal coverage suffer from access issues and waiting lines because demand can exceed supply if there is no volume or cost control.

- Free-market capitalistic health care systems are reeling from spiraling cost and health care disparities. They tend to create a have and have-not, two-tiered system. This is why the United States health care system struggles both with quality and cost. It is a case of Richland versus Poorland with vastly diverging health care outcomes for each and how it played out for Richard and Paul. These gaps in disparity have turned into graves of disparity (44).

- There will be a migration away from extremes of health care delivery, avoiding both the single-payer system on one end of the spectrum and the totally free-market system on the other, moving instead towards some hybrid answer in the middle. Each country will have its own version of doing this to meet its own needs.

- The greatest driving force leading many countries to select their health care systems is a deep cultural belief that the good of the whole exceeds the value of the individual in the system. Such an ethos around solidarity and commitment to quality of care for everyone has tended to guide how such countries have developed their health care systems.

America has wrestled with the ethos outlined in the last point above. Thus, in the next chapter we will dive into how America has tried to find its own unique health care system that reflects the will and spirit of our people, based on our culture's values of autonomy, choice, and self-determination.

Chapter 6

NINE OBSERVATIONS ON WHY AMERICA STRUGGLES WITH HEALTH CARE FOR ALL

In Chapter 5 we compared health care in the United States with that in other nations. We also identified large differences between health care for the rich and the poor within our own country. Let's now ask some basic questions: Are the discrepancies in health care quality available to differing groups of Americans the unavoidable result of our culture? Do we desire a level health care playing field as a basic right for all of our citizens, or do we prefer to keep our have and have-not system? This moral quandary is central to the entire health care debate. To understand this more deeply, let's delve into a few characteristics that define who we are as Americans.

First, it should be noted that most Americans do maintain that they want a more affordable, accessible, fair, and efficient health care system, and actually favor many recent health care reform provisions. A Kaiser Family Foundation poll shows that a majority of U.S. residents support several elements of the health care reform law enacted in 2011 (1). For instance, 86 percent support small business tax credits to help provide health care insurance for employees, 82 percent favor preventive services with no co-payments, 81 percent favor banning insurers from dropping coverage for preexisting medical conditions, and 74 percent favor allowing children to stay on their parents' insurance plans until age 26 (1).

Nevertheless, the fact that we could not achieve even more robust reform does reveal some essential features of America's culture. Let's explore several underlying reasons why America struggles with health care reform. What is it about the American psyche that so polarizes us when such reform is pursued? I'd like to suggest that there are at least nine deterrents in our culture that resist changes to our health care system.

1. THE FEAR OF CHANGE AND UNCERTAINTY

America is a progressive nation, but it also has a conservative undercurrent that fights change. An easy way for reform opponents to block change is to inject fear and confusion; to flood the airways with prophecies of cost, government control, and national debt. Instead of discussing what it means for the good of the country and one's children, the debate is framed around how it would hurt existing health care, warning that "the devil you know is safer than the devil you don't." When painted like this, it is likely that individuals will say no rather than yes. This dynamic affected the health care reform debate, most visibly during the town hall meetings of 2009; especially those organized by the Tea Party movement. There has emerged much anger, fear, and distrust of government meddling, particularly when extending benefits to others might mean costs to us all. This fear has been targeted at the 171 million insured patients against the 50 million uninsured. It is a status quo tactic to say, "I have mine, now you get yours."

Another way fear forestalls change in our health care system is through predictions of "rationing": threats of denied care, long waiting lines, and restricted choices. Keep in mind that all health care rations to some degree. Only when it is done for the wrong reason is it a problem. Actually, the worst case of rationing in our country now is that health insurance plans often deny coverage to individuals for preexisting conditions or drop them when they're sick, exactly when they need it the most. On the other hand, rationing health care based on scientific evidence and efficacy—in other words, does the treatment work or not—can be a good idea. There must be cost effective decisions made based on evidence of treatment effectiveness that will steer wise use of limited resources. We cannot do everything for everyone, and sanity and common sense must enter into the equation in a manner that doesn't create public fear.

2. FAILURE OF RESOURCES

Fear of cost has been one of the boogeymen thwarting health care reform. Let's analyze this a bit. The price of the health care law that stands is $938 billion over 10 years, or about $93.8 billion per year. Recall that our current United States health care spending bill is $2.6 trillion per year. Therefore, an extra $93.8 billion a year to broaden coverage and reform health care represents only 3.6 percent of our nation's annual health care cost. This is a real bargain. Why would we not want to increase our spending by only 3.6 percent to reform health care?

Yet Americans resist anything that is believed to cost them more. We are not willing to pay more in taxes from our hard-earned dollars for anything lacking direct personal value. As mentioned earlier, "pulling one's self up by one's own boot straps" is our motto. Therefore, instead of health care reform being praised as an investment for the greater good of our country, it is seen as a penalty and an increased taxation on the individual. It is hard for us to focus on the larger concept of the greater good when the lens of reality is tightly focused on day-to-day survival at the individual level.

Beyond this, the opposition asserts that health care reform will obviously add large debt to America's bottom line. Actually, the Congressional Budget Office (CBO), the bipartisan accountants of the U.S. Congress, has shown that overall, health care reform will decrease its impact on the national deficit over the next 10 years by $124 billion, and by an additional trillion dollars in the decade after that (2, 3). Remember that the cost of insurance premiums are growing four times faster than wages and our Medicare population will double from 40 to 80 million in the next 15 years. As a consequence, without health care reform the real danger is that the cost to the American economy will be catastrophic. For the good of the

American economy, we cannot fail to act now.

3. INCONSISTENT MESSAGING

With an issue as complex as health care reform, communication is difficult. On one hand, we talk about expanding coverage and ensuring access, and on the other, we talk about cost containment. Is this about health care expansion or is this about health care cost reform? Is this about health insurance reform through regulatory mechanisms or is this about enhancing free-market choices through competition? Each of these messages plays well with certain groups but not well with others. Therefore, when we talk about quality, access, and cost, the message can rapidly become diffused. This helps those who want to oppose health care reform, since they can point in a piecemeal way to these potential inconsistencies to generate fear and misinformation.

Because of the complexity of health care reform and its many moving parts, we've lacked a coherent message to move and inspire the country. Instead of increasing understanding, we've actually contributed to fragmentation and polarization. Unfortunately, President Obama, in his attempt to ensure that health care reform was bipartisan and came from Congress, was unfocused and sporadic in his early messaging and campaigning for health care reform. Now, it should be remembered that when he took office he had two wars to conduct, a financial banking crisis, a tanking American economy, a collapsing auto industry, and a growing unemployment problem to dominate his limited time, but his absence of guidance at a critical time clearly led to the health care reform message being co-opted by those who wanted to undermine health care reform.

Additionally, the power of money to define the argument and preserve the status quo is a key factor in creating inconsistent and fragmented messages. Money not only often controls the agenda, it usually controls the message. This has been the case for as long as we have had health care in this nation. It's not that companies and businesses that make lots of money in health care are composed of malicious people. But it is inevitable that wealth wants to continue to influence the policies, procedures, and laws that are to its benefit. This does drive the question: at what point do our responsibilities and obligations extend beyond our own bounds and reach our communities, our states, and our nation?

What also makes messages confusing is the echo chamber of the public media. We are being polarized by the very rapid cycling of news in our country. Day and night nonstop news, especially through the Internet, blogs, and 24-hour news stations, has created a reverberating, booming echo chamber. This has powerfully amplified division in our country. For any blog or news item to be widely read, it now needs to be memorable and sensational not just fact-based or true. No longer is just news reporting the goal; it is also to create emotion. This has created a dynamic in which many people choose sides, abandon the middle ground, and stop listening to each other. Health care reform finds itself in the crosshairs of this effect. America is very much like a bell-shaped curve with some left-wing and right-wing members on the opposite ends of the curve, but with most people gathered towards the middle. But during battles for viewers that rage in the media, there is a constant barrage of confusion and fear to overcome for those in the middle.

Many have just been too busy to keep up with the health care reform debate. There is so much information concerning coverage, access, cost, and insurance reform that it has been very dizzying for most Americans. In fact, a Kaiser Family Foundation survey found that 55 percent of Americans were confused about health care reform and 56 percent said they do not have enough information to decide (1). If you are uninformed when it comes time to take a stand on health care reform, your natural default is to settle for the status quo. If anybody then adds misinformation or disinformation to increase your confusion, fear, or frustration, then you tend to dig in your heels even more. This can set up a default condition in which people do not want to change health care or the larger health care system. This will be even more likely if it means increased taxation to you as an individual, or if there is any concern you might lose existing coverage and current insurance benefits.

4. FAILURE OF IMAGINATION AND VISION

When our Founding Fathers created the United States of America, they were guided by what we were for, not what we were against. One of our nation's many strengths is that we like to be inspired. We like hope and a vision of a better tomorrow. In this regard, I think we have failed to gather our nation's imagination around the greater good of health care reform. Unfortunately, through special interest groups and politics, the message of inspiration and hope has been watered down by fear and by anger, and by uninspiring messages of cost and what it means to me (and not you). This has made opposition easier than reform.

On this note, although our president and many in Congress have portrayed health care as a greater good for our nation, they have failed to inspire people's imaginations about what the future would look like with and without health care reform. Instead of talking about what we need and what we are trying to build for the good of all, we are wrapped around the axle of what we already have and the inevitable problems of getting from point A to point B. Instead of aspiring toward what we want, we have become hamstrung by what we have.

5. ISSUES DIVIDE US EASIER THAN THEY BRING US TOGETHER

America has been structured in large part in response to what divides our country. When you think about it, our federal government was created with a system of checks and balances to counteract competing forces. Our federal system of the executive, legislative, and judicial branches was formed to ensure that no one part of our government has too much power. This has led to a system of governance in which saying no is much easier than saying yes. This has been a strength but also a weakness for our country. In the last 100 years we have rallied as a nation most strongly during World War I and World War II, and for a brief moment after 9/11. There have been many more events that have polarized us over the years, such as the Civil War, slavery, desegregation, the battle over civil rights, Vietnam, immigration, and abortion. This effect has been magnified by our two-party political system, in which parties take opposing sides like rowdy children playing dodgeball. Although it is good to have choice in our country, it has been hurtful to have it boiled down to simply one versus the other. Unfortunately the reductionism of our two-party system has thrown issues into camps of black and white as opposed to gray. But the real truth is there are shades of gray in most everything, including health care systems, and it may be more beneficial to have multiple parties looking at this challenge in different ways.

America is famously diverse, with many ethnic groups, languages, religions, and lifestyles. This has been good for the youthful vigor of our country. Diversity, however, can create barriers when we try to pull together for the good of everyone's health care. America has always suffered from a certain amount of xenophobia. In contrast, it has been easier for those countries with individuals who are prone to look alike, talk alike, and think alike to declare that health care belongs to all citizens. This is the case in countries such as Denmark, Norway, and Sweden. It is much harder for a country like America. Individual Americans often anguish over extending an open hand to people with health care needs when those people don't look like them, speak like them, believe like them, or act like them. When we try to wrap our arms around health care reform for everyone, too much diversity can be distracting, and can in fact create fissures, fractures, and polarization. This is particularly true when considering the health care needs of illegal immigrants. As a result, recent health care reform bills have been careful to insist that care not be given to those in our country illegally. This has been the case even though one can make a strong case that by including illegal immigrants such noncitizens would actually receive better health care and yet cost America less as a whole.

America spans 50 states, multiple territories, contains more than 312 million people, and encompasses over 3.5 million square miles. As a result, we have lost some of our sense of community. Many drive back and forth to work in cities that are far from where they live. Many people don't know their neighbors. People move across the country and may not live where they grew up or near other family members. The Internet has also contributed to this separateness by downplaying face-to-face communication in favor of distant, asynchronous, electronic communication. This is not all together bad as a new social tool, but it comes at a cost of community identity and a spirit of togetherness and cooperation. This separateness is yet another reason why many do not to want to be a participant in something like health care reform that benefits the greater good, as opposed to simply oneself.

It is a trait in human society to have a pecking order and social classes. America is no different in this regard. There are many ways to stratify people: race, ethnicity, religion, language, or socioeconomic status. There is a belief embedded in the fabric of American culture that those who work harder and succeed should have more of everything, and those that don't should not benefit from the spoils. Therein lies ambivalence when it comes to providing health care for everyone in this country: "It is something that I've been able to achieve, so why can't they?" Or when that question is compounded with: "What do you mean I need to pay more in taxes to cover them?" Or finally, the complaint: "Why should I want my money used to cover them, if that might mean less for me?"

6. CAPITALISM

Our form of government lends itself to the competitive, entrepreneurial spirit. That's good for business. It can become a problem, however, when it comes to health care, surrounding it with a single-minded individualism. How should one answer the question of is it my responsibility to take care of others, especially if those others are not like me, don't work for me, live in different states, and have different cultures and values than I do? Franklin D. Roosevelt said, "The test of our progress is not whether we add more to the abundance of those who have much; it is whether we provide enough for those who have too little." (4) This is a statement that all boats ought to float upward together to at least a certain minimum level. Not that everyone must be the same nor be limited in their opportunities, but that everyone should be entitled to at least a basic amount.

America has become great because of our capitalism and entrepreneurial spirit. It has given us our business, banking, financial, and economic foundation. It has also given us our health care system. Our American health care system is driven to make profit. It is based on volume and fees for services. It is perfectly designed to give us what a capitalistic system will produce: volume, profit, goods, and services. It is designed to generate wealth, not necessarily health. Unfortunately what this has produced in the realm of health care is an expensive, high-cost, inefficient system that often generates mediocre quality health outcomes. It is not paid or rewarded to keep people healthy or to prevent disease from occurring. It is paid and rewarded to do things to people and to generate money. The incentives of capitalism are not always well aligned with health care, and define one of the most important struggles in trying to change our health care system. This is not to say that capitalism and health care cannot be structured to productively coexist. They certainly can. It is just that you have to reward the right things if you want the system to generate health outcomes instead of wealth outcomes.

Health care in the United States, however, is more complicated than the simple notion of capitalism versus socialism. Any unilateral critique of capitalism's effect on health care's availability, quality, or cost would be far too simplistic. The solution most likely does not lie in the two-dimensional dichotomy of capitalism versus socialism, but in a more complex three-dimensional trade-off between these two philosophies and a good dose of what is collectively right for communities, states, and the nation. A middle-ground solution must be found that recognizes the complexities of health care and resides in the sweet spot between the extreme positions of "capitalism or nothing" or "anything but capitalism."

Anything that takes money from one group and gives it to

another, or limits one's ability to freely make money, is an anathema to many Americans. Obviously, companies and businesses that have made a lot of money around health care do not want to lose that ability. They've built up an infrastructure, research and development, and jobs based on that income. Plugging up that financial pipeline becomes a problem. However, one must ask how much is enough? Is it okay instead of making a 6 percent profit to make a 25 percent profit or higher? Is 3 to 4 percent profit acceptable? Similarly, anything that takes money away from individuals or families, through increased taxation or other charges, is seen as a larger negative than a greater good. Instead of everyone getting an equal opportunity to have great health, we see this as an individual issue based on lifestyle, income, personal choices, and behaviors. Phrases such as "keep your hands off my money" when directed at health care reform are indicative of our country's mind-set. I am not saying that it is desirable to pay greater amounts of money in taxation or to have other people take hard earned dollars out of any of our pockets. But at what point does the nation as a whole see this as an investment in our health productivity and excellence, as opposed to being a weight on "my own" personal income?

7. FEAR OF GOVERNMENT CONTROL

Americans have a love–hate relationship with our government. We want it there when it serves us, but at the same time we want it blocked from meddling in our life. We walk a fine line between our government's presence and our government's absence. Our government's involvement with health care is a classic example. In 1965, the government created Medicare and Medicaid to provide both the elderly and the poor basic coverage, because the wealth-based health care system existing at that time left these two important groups of people stranded. We had a lot of people suffering without care because they could not afford it. Nevertheless, at that time Medicare and Medicaid were branded by many as socialism or even communism, and were fought tooth and nail by special interest groups as being anti-American.

We are once again at a crossroads. As before, reform has been branded by opposition forces as inappropriate interference and a government takeover at its worst. The rallying cry of many opposed to health care reform has been, "keep your hands off of my health care," and more ironically, "keep your hands off of my Medicare." It speaks to an irrational fear that the government, through its ineptness, inefficiency, or even bad intent will hurt people or take things away from them. It badly blurs the fine line that must be considered when balancing the common good against basic individual freedoms.

Fearmongers point to Canada, or England and other European countries, and declare that America does not want a health care system like that. Those in this opposition are quick to cart out fears of rationing, of waiting lines, and of massive costs. The truth is, however, that these countries' health care systems are actually running much more efficiently at lower costs, better quality, and with better health care outcomes than in America. Another underappreciated truth is that in America there is more interference imposed on the doctor–patient relationship from private insurance companies than there is from the federal government. No one wants regulation that is out of control and restricts our freedoms. On the other hand, no one wants a totally unregulated system that is a free-for-all, leaving millions of people uncovered and destitute; a system where those with means get everything they need, when they want, and others do not. Or do we? It is a question of balance.

To many in our nation, the federal government (even though it is democratically elected) is just not to be trusted, and this distrust has grown greatly over the last few years. Not only does this extend to accusing the government of being unable to do the right thing efficiently and effectively, but it also asserts that the federal government does not have the right plan or the right reasons. This lack of trust is demonstrated in the willingness of many people to believe that massive health care reform will inevitably affect individual lives in deleterious ways, and this belief is amplified in the echo chamber of the media that spins the facts to enhance viewpoints they are marketing.

8. THE MATURITY OF AMERICA

America is in point of fact a rather young country. We are only 236 years old and have not yet learned some of the lessons of our elder-nation colleagues. Our self-image is of being a young, vibrant, innovative, and competitive country, not an older, secure, and comfortable one. We do not always believe that one of a nation's major responsibilities is to provide certainty and security for the good of the whole, for the good of us. Our focus rather has been on a more vibrant and somewhat narcissistic me. If you will, our country acts much more like an adolescent teenager than it does a mature adult. In many ways we have not truly matured as a country around many of our social issues. This is not all together bad and helps fuel our country's dynamic creativity. However, this lack of social responsibility when applied to health care can create a problem for those in our nation who do not have the means and are not youthful and vibrant. For the poor, for the aged, for the mentally ill, and for those with medical disabilities, the lack of "us" can create a dilemma.

Almost all other industrialized countries have already determined that health care is a basic right and they work hard to ensure that it is available for the greater good of their people. For example, in Germany 81 percent of the Germans believe that equal access is more important than the 18 percent who believe their own access is the best path (5). We in America resist the premise that the greater good is to the whole rather than to the one. It is in that maturational ethos that we as a country struggle with health care reform. For example, many will argue that while people in low-income jobs choose not to buy health insurance because it is too expensive, they as individuals nevertheless spend money on smoking, drinking, and making other bad personal choices, so why is their situation my problem? We as a nation tend to judge whether somebody deserves something or not. There's not a recognition that a society that is well-educated, decently housed, getting enough food, and receiving appropriate health care will be more productive, creative, and less motivated to commit crime. But if these protections were guaranteed, would we not be a more successful nation? Specifically, wouldn't we agree that every individual should have the benefit of health care? In point of fact, many in this nation don't.

9. RUGGED INDIVIDUALISM

The principle of rugged individualism is both a strength and a weakness for America, and is the one principle that most firmly stands in the way of recognizing health care reform as a greater societal good. America is a country of rugged individualists who want autonomy. We are driven by this ethos, even when tackling issues intended to help the country as a whole. Thus, while it makes sense to Americans to have a standing army and a police force to keep us safe for the common good, we struggle when trying to advance the common good for less-visceral issues. For example, education tends to be an area where our country chafes at government involvement (though we have at least become comfortable considering education a basic individual right from kindergarten to 12th grade). Similarly, we wrestle with individual health care as a basic right. Part of the complexity of this issue is the tension between our Judeo-Christian philosophy of "being our brother's keeper" versus the American bedrock aphorism of "pulling oneself up by one's bootstraps." In other words, "I have mine, now you get yours!" This means that instead of helping everyone achieve a certain standard of health so they can maximize their own unique abilities and talents, we question whether health care is really a basic human right to be extended to everyone. Shouldn't it rather be a money-based privilege, not given by the federal government but instead a reward for status and hard work?

This creates paradoxes on several fronts. Ironically, we have no problem accepting health care as an important benefit from employers, but we do challenge such support from our government. To top this off, our government already covers health care for nearly 33 percent of all people under provisions of Medicare, Medicaid, SCHIP, Tricare, VA, Department of Defense, and the Indian Health Services. So what is the big conflict? It is that the symbol of the rugged individualist argues that we not permit government to take over health care and by extension our lives? America is divided on this issue of government involvement. Health care has become the new battleground for individual versus state versus federal control rights. It challenges the deeply held values and ideologies of many.

There are many Americans who believe that providing everyone a basic minimum of health insurance and access to health care is an expansion of the welfare state, and only encourages dependency and laziness in those that do not currently have access to basic health care. It is claimed that this condones a lack of personal accountability and competitiveness; rewarding the jobless. To equate health care to welfare returns us to the essential question, is health care a basic right that should be granted to everyone or not? If it is, then this is not welfare but a basic human right. If it is your perspective that it is not a basic human right, then when given to the less fortunate it can be labeled as welfare. America, for better or worse, seems to be wandering somewhere in between these two views. On a personal level, it is my observation that most people do not want to be dependent or perceived as lazy. What they want is an equal chance to get up off the ground. They are proud and caring, and want to achieve whatever success they can. These are people who want a helping hand, not a handout.

In conclusion, health care reform is a complex issue that strikes at what every individual American personally values. It also asks us to extend an open hand beyond ourselves and our immediate families for the greater good of all. As has been seen in this chapter, there are many factors in conflict. There are the macro forces of politics and special interest groups that desire that the status quo continues for their own self-interest. There are a host of other issues, however, that impact individuals, their families, their communities, and their states. Health care reform has meaning to everyone involved. If the message is not crystal clear that the benefits of health care reform result in a better life for the individual, then it will be a tough sell against the opposing forces that exalt in pointing out how reform may hurt you as an individual. This plays out in fear, misinformation, and a doubt that what you have is really better than what you will receive. That, coupled with our country's ethos, has spawned a multitude of individually minded responses from the citizens of our country.

Trying to change health care for the greater good of this country is challenging. To convince people over the long haul, it will have to be shown how this change will make individual American lives better. The Affordable Care Act will need to demonstrate that cost for health care will be less, quality will be higher, and access more rapid. These things are yet to be clearly proven and the country will be watching closely. Many reasons mentioned above have in the past shepherded many individuals to think that health care is not a basic right. Only when we have formed a majority opinion around the assumption that health care *is* a basic right, will we be able to move forward collectively as a nation to maximize the benefits of health care reform for all. Other countries have been much more successful in their abilities to target their norms around this very important point. America has not. Until we all recognize some of the dynamics that have shaped our American personality and work on cleverly adapting these attitudes to address our problems, health care reform will be accomplished only in half-measures.

Chapter 7

WHO STANDS TO WIN AND LOSE WITH HEALTH CARE REFORM?

Large numbers are often very hard to grasp, and in this chapter, we're going to focus on some enormous numbers indeed. Recall that the annual cost of providing health care in this country is about $2.6 trillion. At 17 percent of the gross domestic product, this is the largest single segment of the nation's entire spending. This figure translates to a cost each year of approximately $8,500 for every man, woman, and child in America. There are many powers that want to keep this system exactly as it is, since it generates large sums of money for a lot of people. While this does help fuel America's economy, at what cost do we provide health care for the people of our nation? As noted in an earlier chapter, America's health care cost per person is two to four times the average spent by the rest of the industrialized world. We pay 40 percent more than the next closest country for a health care system that is more known for treatment than for prevention, and more concentrated on disease and illness than on health and wellness. If channeling vast revenue is the goal, then our system is a powerhouse. However, if good health is the goal, one can easily argue that the system is not well designed.

The American health care system is constructed to generate income in large amounts for individuals and services that do things to people. Therefore, it is not surprising that procedures (imaging, lab work, medications, and patient visits) are done in very large quantities. Volume and quantity in our health care system directly translates to financial gain. It is not unexpected that changing our health care system, which may change the way in which health care is delivered and paid for, will threaten the forces at play in America's largest economic sector. In fact, many would argue that there are 2.6 trillion reasons to leave things just as they are.

President Obama, at the White House Summit on March 5, 2009, forcefully stated two things. First, the current state of our costly health care system, with its mediocre outcomes and 46.7 million uninsured people, is unacceptable to our country. The second was that to move our health care system forward, we as a nation must be willing to sacrifice for the greater good (1). At a fundamental level, almost everyone can agree with these statements. However, accepting possible personal and organizational income changes that result from following these ideals can become quite another story. As James Madison, the fifth president of the United States said, "We are not a government; we are a nation of special interests that run our government." (2) Therefore, the challenge becomes can we all give a little to get a better national outcome for our country's health care system?

America's health care system is full of good people doing good things for the greater good of our country. However, the health care industry's profit-driven forces can be quite catastrophic to our nation's final combined health care price tag. These forces constitute such venerable entities as our nation's hospitals, physicians, insurance companies, pharmaceutical companies, device manufacturers, federal and state governments, nursing homes, home health agencies, dentists, and other institutions and agencies that all have hands in the $2.6 trillion per year health care pot of gold.

Of course, there are counter-forces at play that want to bring some sanity to the cost and accessibility delivered by our nation's health care system. These forces are in the form of such entities as consumer groups, unions, big business, small business, federal and state governments, and our elected leaders. We have an inevitable tension between those who want to keep the health care system just as it is because of its ability to generate wealth, and those that oppose the health care system as it is because of its cost, insurance problems, disparities, access problems, and uneven quality. These are not good or bad people or right or wrong people lined up on either side of this battlefront. They are individuals and groups who are looking at the same conflict but from different perspectives. One group wants to continue the status quo not only for improving people's health but for what it means to the lifestyles and wealth that health care has created in this country. The other group wants to provide a more equitable, affordable, and accessible health care system for the good of the whole.

Changing the revenue stream of the medical-industrial complex does not happen easily, which is why the 2009 health care reform bills and the Accountable Care Act of 2010 were such big deals. They created upheavals that are seismic in scale. Like two tectonic plates pushing against each other, one side wanting to retain the status quo and the other trying to change it, the opposing sides in health care reform have created major fault lines. Unfortunately, you cannot change our health care system—the largest economic sector in the American economy—without creating winners and losers. You cannot change the health care system without fracturing the bonds that are holding it in place. The battleground has become the United States House of Representatives, the United States Senate, the White House, and the media. The battle is also being fought within the hearts and souls of the American people. What is at stake is our will and ability to implement the current new laws, and future laws and policies that alter the terrain of our health care system. This is definitely a shakeup of seismic proportions!

So let's examine in a bit more detail where the United States health care dollar is spent. Since, as the old saying goes, "you can't tell the players without a scorecard," look at Figure 1 to see by category how much of the combined $2.24 trillion spent in 2007 went to each player in the health care industry (3).

Figure 1. 2007 U.S. Health Expenditures

	TOTAL	$2,241,200,000,000
1.	Hospital Care	$696,500,000,000
2.	Physician and Clinical Services	$478,800,000,000
3.	Prescription Drugs	$227,500,000,000
4.	Administration/Net Cost of Insurance	$155,700,000,000
5.	Nursing Home Care	$131,300,000,000
6.	Dental Services	$95,200,000,000
7.	Government Public Health Activities	$64,100,000,000
8.	Home Care	$59,000,000,000

Source: Hartman M, Martin A, et al. Health Affairs 2009;28:1;246-261

HOSPITALS

Hospitals represent the single largest expense within the United States health care system at $696.5 billion per year and 31 percent of national health expenditures and produce over 5 million jobs for America. There are approximately 5,815 hospitals in the United States (4). Hospitals are present in just about every community across this nation, and most have been there for long periods of time. They are there to provide health care services and to be safety nets in their communities. Hospitals are often the largest, or second largest, single employer in a town or city and are very important to the fabric of the communities they serve. Therefore, changes that threaten the income of health care services have far-reaching implications for these hospitals, their employees, and their communities. If health care reform means a healthier nation in which less hospitalization occurs, if more people are actually having less disease, and if there are fewer operations, less imaging, and less diagnostic work, then there is an impact on the size of hospitals, their operations, the number of employees they have, and potentially the economies of their communities. It is with this in mind that hospitals are concerned about what health care reform may mean to them. There has been a lot of lobbying on behalf of America's hospitals to help craft legislation in a way that protects them in the future. One thing is for sure, hospitals will need to evolve their business strategies to continue to deliver multiple beneficial services to their communities and regions.

Hospitals have a lot at stake as we proceed from the Industrial Age into the Information Age. As we do more at the front end of health care to keep people healthy, and as we redirect care to the ambulatory and outpatient sector, hospital-based health care systems have much to be cautious about. As health care becomes more ambulatory-friendly and more primary care-focused (rather than subspecialty, tertiary, and disease-focused), there are major shifts that will occur in delivery models and revenue generation. Unless hospitals move away from being monolithic, large bricks-and-mortar structures that provide the same sort of services they have for the last 100 years and become innovative centers in which they augment prevention, wellness, and streamlined inpatient care, they will struggle under health care reform.

As a reaction to this, hospitals are watching payment reform measures in the Affordable Care Act very carefully. They are looking to preserve as much of the status quo as is possible. However, failing this approach, they are also poised to restructure themselves along the lines of Accountable Care Organizations (ACOs) or other models of care that maintain revenue flow and control. These changes will coincide with possible payment reforms, so that teams of physicians within coordinated care systems may become a new model on which to base patient care. These new models will focus on higher quality, better patient outcomes, and cost savings. In fact, the shared savings model of the Accountable Care Organization will look to split these savings roughly 50/50 between ACOs and insurance payers (Medicare, Medicaid, private insurance companies) that provide this higher quality and cost savings. These ACOs are different than the old managed care models of the 1990s. Figure 2 below compares and contrasts this new ACO model from the old managed care model.

Figure 2. Comparison of Capitation (1990s) Versus ACO (2010s) Models

HMOs/Capitation	Accountable Care
Provider centric	People/patient centric
No consistent system entry point	Primary care/medical home
Fragmented delivery system	High value integrated – delivery system
Only health plans have population based data	Provider system has population based data
Insurance industry driven	Provider driven
Shift risk to PCPs	Shift risk to aligned, integrated system
HMO-driven	Medicare-driven
Financially led	Enhanced business skills of clinicians
Growth Economic Period	Challenging financial climate
Limited patient choice	Enhanced patient choice
Barriers to care	Bridges to care

It is not surprising then to see hospitals buying up doctors' groups and a large number of physicians' practices in order to incorporate these entities into the larger hospital system. This allows hospitals control over how patients flow and how vertically integrated teams can maximally function. Therefore, if in the future payment practice switches to covering episodes of care rather than assigning costs to individual diagnostic codes of care (as in the currently common fee-for-service approach), then hospitals will be situated to control the flow of money. The payment structure will shift from fee-for-service to bundled payments or global payments for these episodes. If you own all the providers along with the facilities that provide the services, then you are in a powerful, self-preserving, and self-sustaining position.

However, if cost of care is decreased mostly by downsizing volume of hospital utilization and by reducing the cost of procedures and imaging, then hospitals will stand to lose money. If the forces at play are also trying to keep people healthy and out of hospitals by providing better primary care in outpatient clinics versus the inpatient hospitals, then revenue streams will also shift or dry up. This has been seen in the trend towards hospitalists (physicians who only care for patients in the hospital) and employing more and more emergency room physicians. With health care reform focusing on keeping patients healthier and out of hospitals and emergency rooms, both of these lines of service will be downsized going forward. If you want to understand how the American health care system works and how change will affect it, all you have to do is follow the flow of money through the health care system. Since hospitals are the largest, single recipient of health care spending, they stand to lose the most in health care reform. Hospitals know they must evolve and the forces of health care reform will hasten this evolution to new entities that are not yet clearly defined or understood.

PHYSICIANS

Physicians and clinical services represent the second-largest expense within the United States health care system at $478.8 billion per year and 21 percent of national health care expenditures. There are approximately 730,800 physicians in the United States (or about 419 Americans per physician) (5). This ranks us second in the world after China for the total number of physicians. In fact, we have more physicians than India, which has a population greater than three times that of the United States. By that standard, America has more than enough physicians. The problem, however, is that America has the wrong mix of physicians. We have many in the tertiary and subspecialty end of the profession who have focused on small, high-end practices. These practices are quite lucrative and turn on providing services centered on high-end subspecialty procedures and imaging that are mainly focused in hospitals or surgical and imaging centers.

We have way too few primary care physicians, particularly in rural areas and the inner city. The reason for this is that they're paid less for their services and our health care system does not incentivize health care, wellness, and prevention as much as it does disease, illness, surgical procedures, and radiologic imaging.

Health care systems currently built on top of large amounts of procedures, interventions, and high-end hospital work will dig in their heels, rather than allow this model to be altered. It is no surprise that the American Medical Association (AMA), which represents the nation's medical specialties of all kinds, has traditionally been against health care reform. The numerous types of physicians represented by the AMA often prevented it from speaking with a collective voice for change due to the impact it would have on its varied physician membership. This had been true of every reform effort involving health care back to 1911. Of note, however, in the 2009–2010 health care reform bills, the leadership of the American Medical Association stood strong for health care change in our nation. This has been a surprise considering its past history, as well as a shock to a certain sub-segment of its more militant, anti-change, status-quo membership. In fact, not dissimilar to the impact of health care reform on our nation and our people, there has been a fracture within the house of medicine due to the impact of health care reform.

Having said this, the more progressive elements of the American Medical Association has formed its tenants of health care change around the following premises:

- Provide health insurance coverage for all Americans.

- Enact health insurance market reforms that expand choice of affordable coverage and eliminate denials for preexisting conditions.

- Assure that health care decisions are made by patients and their physicians, not insurance companies or government officials. Patients and their physicians should also have the right to privately contract without penalty.

- Provide investments and incentives for quality improvement, prevention, and wellness initiatives.

- Repeal the Medicare physician payment formula that will trigger steep cuts and threaten seniors' access to care.

- Implement medical liability reforms to reduce the cost of defensive medicine.

- Streamline and standardize insurance claims processing requirements to eliminate unnecessary costs and administrative burdens.

- Modify anti-trust enforcement policies to empower physicians to implement clinical integration and quality improvement initiatives. (6)

What led the AMA leadership to take this bold, courageous step on behalf of the nation's health care reform? The AMA came to this position as it became clear that the status quo is untenable. The AMA has realized that the cost of our health care system is not fiscally sustainable, and that we must move to a broader, more accessible, higher quality system of coverage for all people of this country. This has not made the AMA leadership or the AMA as a whole popular with all of its members. The physicians of America are good people. They are trying to deliver the best possible health care to the people they serve. However, with the specter of health care reform it brings many fears to many physicians' minds. These fears center on governmental intervention and of being told what they can and cannot do. These fears are of the government dictating to physicians what payments will be for services rendered. These fears bring the concern of a loss of autonomy and individual control in their small businesses and their lives.

In many ways it has caused a fracture line to appear between those who provide primary care services and those who provide subspecialty services. This by no means has been uniform, but it has set up contention between the primary care community and the subspecialty community when trying to achieve health care reform. I have had many conversations with my subspecialty colleagues at the American Medical Association and elsewhere, and I will be the first to admit that they have stood strongly behind the principles of the patient-centered medical home (PCMH) and of the need for an expanded primary care workforce, with better pay for primary care physicians. However, many in the association have been very adamant that although they will advocate and help America achieve these things for the greater good, they will fight to the death if you try to take one penny from their pocket.

This dynamic has triggered tension among physicians. Since physicians represent the second largest group, they also stand to lose money in health care reform. Subspecialist physicians who engage in costly high-end procedures and radiologic imaging will most likely face reductions than those in specialties that do not. But underneath all of this, the AMA and the physicians of America do care about health care reform. The sign of this is that in June 2011 the AMA again stepped forward and supported the "individual mandate" that requires all U.S. citizens to have health insurance. This was an important proclamation that America's largest physician organization had taken a stand on the need for health care reform.

PHARMACEUTICAL MANUFACTURERS

The third-largest recipient of U.S. health expenditures, representing about $227.5 billion per year (10 percent of national health expenditures), is the prescription drug industry. If you have a disease (and sometimes even if you don't), you can easily be convinced by the myriad of television commercials hocking "Medication X" that it is the latest miracle drug for you. When people have diseases and illnesses, it is good for business in the pharmaceutical industry. They have developed medications to help people with these diseases to continue to live productive and relatively healthy lives. However, as we move towards a system that is more focused on the front end of medicine, with wellness, prevention, and disease control, the pharmaceutical companies' income will decrease. The concept is simple: better health, less medications; more disease, more medications. Less medication use would be the goal of a healthier nation. If we can work on what causes 40 percent of deaths in this country, we will decrease the amount of medications needed to treat hypertension, hyperlipidemia, diabetes, and the ravages of smoking, alcohol, and obesity. We will always need medications for those people who do develop these problems. But there will be a downsizing in the volume of those services, just as there will be a downsizing in the number of hospitals needed, the number of specialty physicians required, and eventually the quantity of pharmaceutical medications that will be needed to treat these particular problems.

There are many pharmaceutical companies in the United States, but part of what health care reform will do is allow importation from other countries of lower-priced, competitive medications and encourage the use of larger amounts of generic medications. This of course threatens our domestic pharmaceutical companies who have in good faith invested a lot of time, energy, and research and development money to offer new drugs, not for only our country, but for the rest of the world. Having a healthier nation is quite frankly bad for their business. This could hurt both their profitability and jeopardize their ability to continue to do good things for our country and the world. This result could occur if their profit margins changed drastically and fewer resources were directed at research and development of new medications.

Additionally, the period during which a pharmaceutical company has an exclusive patent right to market their medication without competition (which now is seven years) has an effect on the company's ability to recoup the money already invested on research and development. Herein lies the rub for pharmaceutical companies:

how will health care reform threaten their continued stability and solvency in an even more competitive world marketplace? This matter is being highlighted by a new class of drugs known as "biologics," for which the length of time granted for exclusive patent rights became part of health care reform. Biologics are medicinal products created by biologic processes versus chemically synthesized processes. Biologics can include such things as medications, vaccines, gene therapy, living cells and therapeutic proteins. An example of a biologic would be penicillin, a famous antibiotic discovered by Sir Alexander Flemming that was made during a biologic process from *Penicillium fungi.* The pharmaceutical industry, in its effort to gain some control of the seismic changes caused by health care reform, wanted to extend patent protection to 12 years for new medications. This longer patent period, free from competition, allows them the financial incentive to discover new medicines and recoup their research and development costs that can be important for the future of health care.

HEALTH INSURANCE COMPANIES

The health insurance industry is one of the largest segments of health care, and one that needs reform. There are approximately 1,280 health insurance companies offering hundreds of thousands of different policies across this country. They represent the fourth-largest recipient of U.S. health care spending, grossing $155.7 billion per year and representing 7 percent of national health expenditures (3). There are five large health insurance companies that have cornered most of the market in the health insurance industry: Aetna, Cigna, Humana, United Healthcare, and WellPoint. In addition, the Blue Cross/Blue Shield Association includes many state and regional plans under various names.

The health insurance industry has been exempt from anti-trust competition since the McCarran-Ferguson Act of 1948, resulting in very unfavorable competitive pricing. Thus, health insurance industry reform became a large part of what was embedded in the health care reform bills of 2009 and 2010, and eventually in the Affordable Care Act. This was driven by the large profitability of insurance companies that harvest ever-growing insurance premiums from both big and small businesses, as well as from individual American's pockets. It was also coupled with the fact that there is growing disillusion with health insurance companies that drop coverage for the seriously ill, discriminate against patients with preexisting conditions, charge exorbitant out-of-pocket expenses such as deductibles or co-pays, and provide no, or minimal, cost sharing for preventive care. Other consumer protection initiatives that led to health insurance reform are stopping gender discrimination (for women's health-related issues, such as having babies), eliminating caps on total coverage, guaranteeing insurance renewal, and extending coverage for young adults under their parent's policy. In this environment, health insurance companies stand to lose ground if more of what they charge for is administrative overhead instead of paying for clinical and hospital services. They must focus more on paying for health care services rather than denying reimbursement for the health care services that people need.

One can easily argue that health insurance is good for those who have it, but that's only true if it targets the customer's best interest and with health as the main focus. However, many health insurance plans come from for-profit companies in which stockholders stand to gain if the insurance company makes money. In every other industrialized country, insurance companies exist to pay health care bills. That is their function. In our country, insurance companies pay for health care bills as a means to an end: to make profit for their shareholders. This is why many in Congress believed a Public Plan Option was needed. The Public Plan Option was aimed at creating a federal health insurance program that would compete on the open market with private insurance companies. The creation of this option would allow another large, competitive health insurance company at the national level to provide expanded coverage at competitive costs. It was envisioned that this government-run health insurance company would compete with insurance companies and would lead to more people being covered. It was intended to drive competitive health insurance reform.

As can be imagined, the creation of a government-run, competitive health insurance company is something that frightens America's health insurance industry. The Public Plan Option as seen through the lens of the health insurance companies is a massive government takeover of medicine. By out-competing these companies on price and possibly product, the fear is that the government, using economy of scale and administrative efficiency, will capture their clients. They see it as unfair competition and an unlevel playing field, directly threatening their solvency. This was perceived by the health insurance industry as ultimately decreasing people's choices by potentially driving private health insurers out of business. To many, the boogeyman of a government-run health insurance system lurks under the Public Plan Option. Conversely, others see a government-sponsored health insurance program as something that expands coverage to more patients, provides more consumer and employer choices, and raises a challenge to the health insurance industry to provide better service for people at lower costs. In fact, the only thing that kept the health care insurance industry at the table was that the Affordable Care Act was promising to provide new expanded health insurance coverage to 32 million of the 50 million uninsured. This would be a new source of volume for them and was the only way they were going to give up on a pure experience rating model that used preexisting conditions, rescissions, denials of care, and annual and lifetime caps on how much they would pay for health care. Because of this volume surge of 32 million new people into the health insurance system, the health insurance industry was willing to play in order to gain so many new insured people.

NURSING HOME CARE

There are approximately 16,100 nursing homes in the United States. This provides 1.7 million beds with an occupancy rate of 86 percent (7). There are 1.5 million nursing home residents with an average length of stay of 835 days (7). Nursing homes rank fifth in the amount of health care dollars spent per year. This amounted to approximately $131.3 billion in 2007 and 6 percent of national health care expenditures. As the number of elderly Americans rapidly increases, nursing homes become an even larger health care market. Nursing homes can even rival small hospitals as being the largest employer in small rural towns. The forces at play at the front end of health care reform want to keep people healthier and living independently at home as long as possible, and in fact want to decrease nursing home utilization. At the same time, other forces want to produce more efficient, costly, high-quality nursing home care as part of the health care reform bills. Such legislation is very important not only to the nation, but to the states in particular, since most nursing home costs are born by the state once a patient can no longer afford care. It is a sad statement that in our country people must go financially bankrupt before state Medicaid will kick in and pay for nursing home care. Therefore, overhaul and reform in the nursing home industry becomes important.

The number of Medicare-aged individuals will double from 40 million to 80 million Americans in the next 15 years. That coupled with the fact that people are living longer and living sicker sets up a ticking time bomb. With the fastest growing segment of our population by decade being those over 100 years of age, you can see the problem. Where are all these people going to be cared for, and by whom? Most patients do not want nursing home care. They would like to maintain an active life in the comfort of their own home with their independence. Long gone are the days, however, when multiple generations of families lived in the same community and would care for their aging parents and grandparents who were still living in their own homes. Thus, moving elderly parents into a family member's home has become quite common. When care can no longer be easily provided in the home and independence no longer easily accomplished, nursing homes and other community-assisted living centers become viable alternatives. Keep in mind that 95 percent of those over age 65 do not live in nursing homes (8). Most live in their own homes, relative's homes, or other community-assisted living centers. But even 5 percent of 80 million people results in 4 million people living in nursing homes, which exceeds the total available nursing home capacity by 235 percent.

Finding the right balance between keeping people healthy, at home, and functionally independent versus accommodating those that need care at high-quality, safe, clean, and accessible nursing homes will become critical over the next 20 years. Good primary care, ambulatory clinics, wellness and prevention programs, and viable community and home care must be quickly developed. In order to reform elderly health care and control costs we must create alternatives to expensive nursing home care. We must keep people in the community and functional longer. If people do end up in nursing homes, then the cost of that care must become less expensive if this is to be sustainable over the long run. Therefore, nursing homes are in a position to lose from health care reform, since reform forces will want to reduce the need for people to live in nursing homes; and if they do need this sort of care, that it is of both higher quality and lower cost. Conversely, nursing homes also stand to gain from the sheer volume of aging Americans.

DENTAL CARE

There are about 141,900 dentists in America. Of these, 120,200, or 85 percent, are general dentists (9). Dental care in America represents about $95.2 billion of expenditures per year and 4 percent of national health expenditures. This is a part of health care reform that has not been discussed much publicly. However, I will tell you that the three areas of overall health care improvement that must be enacted for us to be a healthier nation are the following: 1) primary care; 2) mental health care; and 3) dental care. Our nation struggles in particular with a have and have-not dental care system. We must expand people's dental health care coverage, and there must be appropriate incentives for our nation's dentists to see patients with this coverage. The dentists in our country become key players by serving more people and by leading teams of dental health care providers to maximize our nation's dental health. We do a relatively poor job with ensuring oral and dental health care for all in our country. We must lower barriers to dental and oral health and pay for this care accordingly. The two most visible signs of a patient's socioeconomic status from a health care perspective are their body habitus (being obese or not) and the status of their teeth. Those with means typically have better dental health care and access to better food sources to prevent dental caries and obesity. Those without means have poorer dental health and tend to be more obese.

HOME CARE

Home health care represents about $59 billion per year in U.S. health care expenditures, and is eight on the list of health care spending at 2.6 percent of national health expenditures. This will be a market that will gain as health care reform becomes more mature. If we use our health care system to decrease hospitalizations and nursing home care, then the location where people will achieve more cost-effective and satisfying care will ideally be in the community and their home. A shift of care into the home health sector could very much help bend the cost curve of health care downward from higher cost institutions such as emergency rooms, hospitals, and nursing homes. Home health care agencies should stand to be net winners as health care reform marches forward. For this to happen, there must exist an interlinked, high-quality health care system that integrates primary care and specialist physicians, along with community providers and home health care agencies. The linking of patients, families, physicians, nurses, and other providers (bridged by emerging technologies of home computers and data devices that communicate through television or the internet) can provide ongoing care and monitoring in ways that will keep patients healthier and away from physicians' offices, the emergency room, or hospitals. There are a myriad of these community agencies and providers, technologies, and services. These agencies will only expand with time as the demand dictates and as money nurtures their growth. Another true source of power in the home care environment is women. As we mentioned earlier, the largest single decision-making authority in our nation are not doctors, nurses, hospitals, insurance companies, or pharmaceutical companies. They are the women of the home: moms, wives, and daughters of aging parents. The women in families have a very important role to play in health care reform. They need to be given the tools and the resources to interact online and with their trusted primary care physicians and their practice teams to make informed medical decisions about their families that maximize health and minimize disease. This is a whole new frontier in health education and the extension of proactive health care into the homes of America.

NURSES AND ADVANCED PRACTICE NURSES

There are approximately 2.6 million registered nurses (RNs) in the United States and as such, makes up the largest part of the health care workforce in our nation (10). There are three typical paths to become a RN: a bachelor's degree, an associate's degree, or a diploma from an approved nursing program. Approximately 60 percent of RNs work in hospitals.

Advanced practice nurses consist of clinical nurse specialists, nurse-midwives, nurse anesthetists, and nurse practitioners. The advanced practice nurses require a master's level degree. In addition to these 2.6 million RNs there are 750,000 licensed practical nurses (LPNs) and 480,000 medical assistants (MAs).

Together this nursing workforce will be critical in caring for America. There are currently shortages of nurses across America, especially in certain geographic and rural locations. Nurses' roles will become more important to the future health care system of America. They are excellent team members and will play larger roles in the community, ambulatory, and outpatient clinical settings. Their roles in the patient-centered medical home, home health care, and non-hospital settings will become increasingly important. The reason for this growing role is because of their competitive salaries, team orientation, good communication skills, and relationships with patients. This increases their value in the future health care system and as such they will stand to gain with ongoing health care reform. As I have said before, every American citizen should be afforded a doctor *and* a nurse; not a doctor *or* a nurse. Doctors and nurses need to redouble their efforts to work together for the good of our patients and our communities. With the movement away from hospital-centered care towards community-based care, the workforce of RNs needed in hospitals will shrink from 60 percent being in hospitals to only about 40 percent being in hospitals.

DEVICE MANUFACTURERS

There are approximately 17,200 device manufacturers in the United States (11), producing high-end, technological products from hip and joint replacement devices to stints for coronary arteries, and everything in between. These valuable devices have allowed people to live longer, higher-quality lives. All of these products are expensive, but there is no question they are important when appropriately used and needed. As America wades through health care reform with the goal of becoming a healthier nation, ideally these devices will be needed less. The decreased use of these devices should result from improved front-end health care and health promotion producing healthier, more functional people with less need for artificial knees, artificial hips, insulin pumps, coronary artery bypass stints, and chronic renal and peritoneal dialysis devices. Also, the emergence of evidence-based research will start to shine a light on which of these products truly increase the quality and quantity of life, and at what cost. There will always be a need by people for these products, ideally just less often. Therefore, as we lower the cost of health care by keeping people healthier—avoiding the need for such devices—these companies will stand to downsize. Alternatively, they will consolidate to reduce the costs of their devices through an economy of scale. With the movement of health care more into the community and away from hospitals, operating rooms, and emergency rooms, the medical device companies will develop more cost-effective devices that will link patients care in their homes. This is where health care is headed and where healthier people will reside.

CONSUMER GROUPS

Consumer groups also have a large stake in the current health care reform battle. These entities represent large numbers of patients (for example, the AARP has approximately 38 million members). Other consumer organizations such as the Alzheimer Association, the American Diabetes Association, Families USA, the National Partnership for Women & Children, and the National Consumer League all have issues of great consequence in the health care reform debate. These organizations will push for gains through health care reform to ensure that their members have better access to more affordable and timely health care of higher quality, lower cost, and greater value. It will be a real plus for these organizations to be on the side of health care reform, as this will be perceived of as a benefit by the majority of their members (as long as the cost can be controlled and it does not jeopardize their access). Advocating for people's health, happiness, prosperity, and independence are good things and should increase membership.

UNIONS

There are approximately 25,350 unions in the United States (12). Unions also stand to gain with health care reform, since more of their members will then have sustainable, affordable health care. This will be seen as a definite benefit of union membership if the union can help their members achieve better health care. Unions have intuitively understood that there is strength in numbers and in solidarity. If all are helped, then all have chances for success.

Unions inherently rely on the collective voice being louder than the individual voice.

BIG BUSINESS ORGANIZATIONS

There are approximately 5,600 businesses in the United States with more than 1,000 employees (13). There are 913 firms with over 10,000 employees. Firms with over 1,000 employees represent only 0.1 percent of the over 5.7 million businesses in the United States. Health care reform is a big deal to the big businesses of our country. The reason is simple: they are going broke on health care costs. Big businesses cannot compete on the world market when large sums of money are being spent on their employees' health care. As suggested in an earlier chapter, this is why General Motors' health care cost is more expensive than the steel it purchases, and why the cost of health care at Starbucks is higher than the cost of coffee it purchases. Health care costs are a major factor in how businesses operate. Therefore, big business has been an advocate of major health care reform in terms of what it means to its expenditures for employee health. Health care reform will help big business' bottom line, in addition to ensuring that its employees have a quality health care system. An added advantage will be to produce a healthier workforce, improving productivity and profitability. Therefore, big business stands to gain from health care reform. In fact, the Patient-Centered Primary Care Collaborative (PCPCC), founded in 2006 by IBM in conjunction with the American Academy of Family Physicians (AAFP) and the American College of Physicians (ACP), aimed at helping transform the United States health care system into a more robust and viable primary care system (14). IBM, under the leadership of Paul Grundy, MD, and Martin Sepulveda, MD, has been instrumental in galvanizing a coalition of over 1,000 participating members from Fortune 500 big businesses, consumer groups, unions, physician organizations, and insurance companies, amongst others to advocate together for the importance of primary care and the primacy of the patient–physician relationship as the heart of health care (14).

The IBM case is a riveting story of why we need health care

reform in the United States. IBM is a multinational organization with approximately 485,000 employees, 1.6 million people if you count family members and retirees, in over 170 countries around the world. It spends approximately $2 billion per year on health care, $1.3 billion of that in the United States. IBM found that its employees received better-quality and lower-cost care in every industrialized country outside of the United States. It wasn't that the physicians or hospitals were worse in the United States. It was that the system of health care was poorer in the U.S. than elsewhere in the world where they had employees. When IBM analyzed why this was the case, they found that it was the lack of a primary care infrastructure in the U.S. compared to other industrialized countries that was at the root of the problem. The lack of coordination and integration of health care, which are fundamentals of primary care, were being amplified by the fragmentation, redundancy, and reduplication of tests and procedures that are the hallmarks of subspecialty care. It was this fundamental recognition of the dysfunction of our health care system that led IBM to rally other big business partners such as Microsoft, Google, Exxon, Walmart, and over 1,000 others to merge with physician organizations, health insurance companies, consumer groups, unions, and others to form the Patient-Centered Primary Care Collaborative. They did so in an effort to try to resolve the fundamental primary care problem in our health care system, and to help our nation achieve a higher-quality and higher-value system at a lower cost.

SMALL BUSINESS ORGANIZATIONS

There are approximately 4.8 million small businesses in the United States with less than 10 employees. This represents about 84 percent of all businesses in our country. If you include businesses with less than 100 employees, this becomes 98 percent of all businesses in the United States (15). Small business organizations can experience mixed results from health care reform. On one hand, it is good for small business organizations to have the benefit of more affordable health care insurance for their employees. This helps ensure a healthier workforce and better profitability for its business. On the other hand, if businesses are small enough that they do not have health insurance for employees, this is a new expense line for the business. With the new provisions of health care reform, this may result in small businesses needing to step up to the plate to pay for health insurance for their employees. Therefore, health care reform for small businesses carries pros and cons. To protect small businesses, provisions were put in place so that health insurance reform would not inadvertently hurt them.

FEDERAL GOVERNMENT

Health care reform for the federal government is a definite gain. The reason is that it allows the nation to better control cost. Additionally, health care reform allows broader coverage, which will decrease health care disparities, flatten out quality gaps in care, and increase access to needed and timely health care. It also focuses care on prevention, wellness, and timely chronic disease management. The reason the federal government endorses health care reform is that it will result in a healthier nation, and let's face it, healthier people cost less than sick people. In parallel, these reforms tend to restrain the cost of fragmented, nonintegrated health care, which is demanding exorbitant amounts of money to fund Medicare and Medicaid programs from the federal government. The federal government with its current administration is assuming a large responsibility for the overall health care of its people. Therefore, designing a system that ensures quality health care for the nation at reasonable cost is a win for the federal government. The hazard for the federal government in attempting to transform our health care system was that it was accused of trying to gain too much control. It was even accused by the right-wing Tea Party faction of being socialistic and communistic. Therefore, the downside of health care reform for the federal government is some loss of trust and further polarization in America on health care.

STATE GOVERNMENTS

Health care reform is a mixed blessing to state governments. On one hand, it is a good thing for more of a state's citizens to have timely, affordable health care. On the other hand, since Medicaid programs are both a state and federal government responsibility, there may be greater expenditures needed from both as health care reform expands Medicaid coverage and children's health insurance programs. As a result, there may be an increased state cost to fund state Medicaid programs. Additionally, some states claim that federal mandates on required health insurance ownership for individuals are unconstitutional. This has played out in the legislatures of 26 states (16) and should not be taken lightly. The issue of the individual mandate will be heard by the Supreme Court in early 2012 with their final ruling coming out in the summer of 2012. The issue for these states is the belief that there should not be mandates for individual health insurance, that no one should be forced to purchase a product like health insurance if they do not want to. The problem is, however, if you cannot require everyone to have health care coverage, you cannot stop the cost of care for the uninsured from being shifted onto the premiums of the insured. This also leads to people not receiving lower cost wellness and preventive care and timely chronic disease management. Without this care, more expensive back-end care in emergency rooms, hospitals, and subspecialists once again pops up.

If states believe that mandated health insurance is unconstitutional, it then puts a major crimp in achieving universal health care coverage. To this end, states have enacted legislation to sue the federal government over the passage of health care reform. This is sad to me, quite honestly. Instead of giving health care reform a chance and trying to make it work, this becomes a political statement. These 26 states are in the process of suing the federal government over the unconstitutionality of mandating an individual to purchase health insurance as a state's rights issue.

REPUBLICANS

Health care reform is a good thing for Republicans in helping the citizens of their states to have healthier, more productive lives. However, at a fundamental level, Republicans are disturbed by the growing costs, growing deficit, and growing power of the federal government. Additionally, the Democrats orchestrated health care reform, which was seen as a negative by the Republicans. Unfortunately, health care reform has become more about politics than it is about policy. The inability of the Republicans to stop the Democrats from passing the Affordable Care Act was feared by the Republicans to become a major negative during the 2010 midterm elections. Therefore, messages were framed to confuse, anger, and frighten many Americans about the changes and their costs. In order to stop the Democrats from taking credit for health care reform, Republicans stood unanimously against it.

History has been pretty clear about what happens when a large Democratic social program passes. The passage of the Social Security Act represents such an example. With the passage of this popular program in 1935 the Democrats held the presidency of the United States for 17 years. This historical point has not been lost on the Republicans. Therefore, they have not wanted to have the Democrats win on health care reform. The Republican Party thus became the party of "no!" for reform. With the pendulum swing of power in the 2010 midterm elections in favor of the Republicans, this set up a more polarized and divisive Congress that now needs to implement (or impede, defund, and delay) various provisions and the appropriation of money for the Affordable Care Act. This led to the House of Representatives approving the Repealing the Job Killing Health Care Law Act in January 2011. This largely symbolic vote (as the Senate would not pass this nor the president agree to this) was viewed by the GOP leaders as a "promise kept." The rancor and polarization has only continued and grown, with the Republican mantra being to repeal and replace instead of to refine and refocus. It also sets up a high-stakes poker game for the 2012 presidential election, where if the nation elects a Republican president much can be done to dismantle the Affordable Care Act. This is why health care reform is a major political issue in the 2012 presidential election.

DEMOCRATS

Health care reform was seen by the Democrats as a win for the most part. They were the party in power, and were able to bring about this reform. Not only should this result in a healthier country with more controlled cost, but the Democrats were able to succeed when others had failed. This ideally should have helped them in the 2010 midterm elections since they were able to say that they were responsible for getting health care reform accomplished. However, since the Republicans were able to more skillfully communicate a message that this was not good for America—based on warnings about costs, deficits, and governmental control of health care—health care reform was seen as uniformly negative by many Americans (many more were just simply baffled and confused). This then became a debacle for the Democrats in the 2010 midterm elections, with many Democrats being swept out and many Republicans swept into office.

That is why the politics of health care reform are now so important and why this has superseded the actual policies and specific provisions of health care reform. The Republican strategy to stall health care reform and to portray it as being bad for America because of its "cost" and "big government" has become how health care reform is commonly debated. Only time will tell which strategy and which portrayal of reality will be the most accurate for our nation over the long haul. The presidential election of 2012 is critical to the future of the Affordable Care Act and other health care reform efforts for our nation. If President Obama is reelected to the presidency, then the implementation of the Affordable Care Act will continue. If he is not reelected, many provisions will change or stop. But either way, health care reform must take place for the best long-term interest of America. Both parties recognize this important fact. The question is how and on what, and whose, time table. Which ideology will prevail—repeal and replace or refine and refocus. The presidential election of 2012 will determine which party will call many of the future shots about the direction and rate of change of the Affordable Care Act and further health care reform.

PRESIDENT BARACK OBAMA

President Obama was elected on a platform of reforming health care, education, and energy. With the incredible roller-coaster ride around reforming our health care system President Obama has not shied away from this challenge. The efforts to reform health care have not been perfect and the messaging has not been as clear and simple as needed, but nothing of this magnitude and complexity was going to be clear, simple, and easy. With the initial derailing of health care reform by the Massachusetts election of Scott Brown (R-Massachusetts) and losing the Democratic supermajority, it was truly up in the air as to what the final result of health care reform in our nation would be. Obama personally led the charge to get health care passed. A moment in time came when the president believed that the passage of this health care reform bill was more important than his serving a second term as president of the United States. Because of this, most of the Democratic component of Congress delivered on health care reform.

However, President Obama's fellow Democrats were decidedly hurt in the midterm elections of 2010, in part due to the denigration of health care reform by the Republicans. Much of this had more to do with the economy than health care itself, but the American people definitely did display global displeasure at the polling booths about America's direction and politics in general. Immediately after the midterm elections, Obama and the Democrats calculated that if the Republicans stopped the health care reform drive at the one yard line, and nothing came from this effort, it would have been a loss that would define the rest of his presidency. But even with the eventual successful passage of the reform bills during the lame-duck congressional session, there were losses and heavy prices to be endured. The content of the bills and the eventual law were greatly watered down compared to President Obama's and the Democrats' initial vision of health care reform. Sacrifices were made both in terms of policy and politics to get any health care reform accomplished.

Therefore, on balance there were wins and losses for President Obama on health care reform. One thing that must be conceded—he saw that health care reform needed to be accomplished, not because we "should" but because we "must." Only time will sort out how this health care legislation will change America, and if Obama can truly unite a terribly divided and fragmented Congress and American people around health care reform. There must be compromise and negotiation for our nation to move forward. America is now going to discover exactly how capable and skillful a leader President Obama is (or is not). His bid for reelection in 2012 will be the single most pivotal and critical determinant around the success of the Affordable Care Act in the foreseeable future. If reelected, progress will continue. If not reelected, much will falter.

THE PEOPLE OF AMERICA

The people of America are very confused about health care reform. This is because of intense political lobbying and debates, misinformation, and outright lies that have been painted around health care change. Americans are wondering at a very fundamental level what is in the health care reform law for them and their family? Will this help them or cost them more? Will it raise their taxes? If they have health care coverage already why should they pay more for some stranger who can't afford it or who doesn't try to stay healthy? Will this law lower their premium? Will their son with hemophilia who has exceeded his lifetime cap on costs, now be covered again? Will their daughter with preexisting medical conditions be able to afford a reasonably priced health insurance plan? Will their nephew with mental illness get health insurance? Can we as a nation afford to do this when our economy is tanking and unemployment is around 8 to 9 percent?

These are fundamental questions in the short term. However, in the long term, health care and health insurance reform are critical for Americans, if for no other reason than to control the cost of health care that already sucks $1 out of every $6 in our economy into the black hole of our health care system. This becomes $1 out of every $4 in 2025, and $1 out of every $2 in 2082. If for no other reason than for cost control, we must enact health care reform now, or every future generation will be pulled into this black hole. Our health care system is dragging our country into economic disaster. It will bankrupt our nation. If you will, it is as if we are all on an airplane that is on an altitude-losing trajectory, surrounded by a landscape of rising terrain. We are doomed to crash unless we change the airplane's trajectory.

An advantage of health care reform is the broadening of coverage to more people, so that there is less shifting of unpaid bills of the uninsured onto insurance premiums for employers, employees, states, and the federal government. Also, health care reform results in people getting more prevention and wellness introduced into their health care earlier, aiding them to cumulatively live healthier, more productive lives. Perhaps one of the biggest things it will give Americans is peace of mind. Americans can rest assured that they will not lose their health insurance if they lose their job, change their job, or develop health care problems that might otherwise deny them coverage. Americans will have insurance plans with affordable premiums. Therefore, it will create a permanent safety net for health care for the good of the people of this country. This will have immediate effects on decreasing personal bankruptcies and allow people an opportunity to achieve their maximum potential.

Additionally, health care reform will start to expand the health care workforce and give each American a personal physician with whom they can establish a trusting relationship. Educating such physicians, who lead teams of providers to look after the patient's best interests by concentrating on that patient as a person, is exactly what America's health care system must do. Allowing primary care physicians to connect the dots of health care—to know when and when not to use the system for the good of the patient—will drive reform forward. This team responsibility between the patient and his or her personal physician is what our nation must demand in order to restore health to health care and move beyond a reactive system of disease or injury care. At the end of the day, health care reform will benefit the health of the people of this nation, just as it has in every other industrialized nation, and as it already has for elderly patients on Medicare and our poor and disabled on Medicaid in our own country. We must see beyond what this means to us as individuals and see more of what it means to us as a whole. The people must step forward collectively and continue to push for, and demand, a better health care system.

SUMMARY

In summary, this chapter points out the many forces at play in our $2.6 trillion per year health care system. This large medical-industrial complex has much to be proud of in terms of its innovation and high-end, complex health care given to people in need. However, it is exactly those same issues of high costs, overutilization, and volume-driven incentives that have exploded our overall cost of health care. It underscores the tremendous revenue-generating power of American medicine.

Health care reform is hard to accomplish. Those that have it good in this system will resist change. Those advocating for the greater good will face forces against which they must stand strong if they wish to change the status quo. It is why President Obama—and a majority of those in Congress—boldly stepped forward to say that we must reform our health care system; that, for the good of America, everyone must be willing to give, if we want to achieve a sustainable health care system for our future (1). Time will tell exactly how much we as a nation are ready to do to get a better functioning, sustainable health care system for all.

Chapter 8

THE SIX PILLARS OF HEALTH CARE REFORM

We have journeyed to a point in our discussion where we must move on from our view of America's history and its dysfunctions in health care to a closer study of the blueprint used most recently to reform it. What are the pillars that sustain this reform? To do this, we need to take a look at what the health care reform efforts of 2009 and 2010 were all about. But to gain some perspective on what shaped the outlines of the health care reform bills in the House and Senate at the beginning of 2009, we need first to understand four events which set the stage for what would be some of the major content in the health care bills that would later be debated in Congress.

EVENT 1: CALL TO ACTION HEALTH REFORM 2009, SENATE FINANCE COMMITTEE CHAIRMAN MAX BAUCUS (D-MONTANA)

In November 2008, shortly after President Barack Obama's election, the chairman of the Senate Finance Committee, Max Baucus (D-MT), stated: "I believe it is the duty of the next Congress to reform America's health care system. In 2009, Congress must take up and act on meaningful health reform legislation that achieves coverage for all Americans, while also addressing the underlying problems in our health system. The urgency of this task has become undeniable." (1) Since the Senate Finance Committee oversees Medicare spending and since Medicare drives much of the health care costs in the United States, this was undeniably a "call to action." It was a major step toward health care reform and put the first chip on the table, pushing both Congress and the American public into health care reform debate. Senator Baucus' health reform proposals centered on three major categories. One by one, these categories are:

1. Ensuring health coverage for all Americans. (1)

- Create the Health Insurance Exchange to offer affordable coverage to all Americans. Provide a marketplace in which to compare and purchase health care insurance. All the companies on the exchange would be precluded from denying coverage to people with preexisting conditions.

- Provide subsidies to families and small businesses that cannot afford health insurance.

- Eliminate racial and ethnic health care disparities.

- Create an expanded Medicare buy-in plan for patients aged 55 to 64.

- Phase out the two-year waiting period for Americans with disabilities.

- Create access to Medicaid for all Americans living below poverty.

- Expand the Children's Health Insurance Program (CHIP) to cover children with family incomes below 250 percent of the federal poverty level.

- Provide increased funding for the Indian Health Service (IHS) for Native Americans and Alaska Natives.

- Mandate that all individuals purchase health care coverage.

- Require that employers that do not provide employee health care coverage contribute to a fund to help cover the uninsured. There were exceptions for small businesses in this provision.

- Focus first on prevention and wellness rather than diseases and treatment. The uninsured would be given a "Right Choices" card that would ensure they had basic access to prevention services recommended by the United States Preventive Services Task Force.

- Provide preventive services to all patients on Medicare, Medicaid, and CHIP, and all plans in the Health Insurance Exchange with little or no co-payment.

2. Improving health care quality and value. (1)

- Revalue and strengthen primary care and chronic care management. Fix the Medicare physician payment formula (sustainable growth rate—SGR).

- Use comparative effectiveness research to inform health care providers as to the best possible decisions for the patient's welfare.

- Use of health information technology by physicians to provide quality reporting and evidence-based decision making.

- Reinvest in the health care workforce to increase the number of primary care physicians.

3. Achieving greater efficiency and sustainable financing. (1)

- Eliminate excessive spending.

- Detect and eliminate fraud waste and abuse in public programs.

- Decrease overpayments to private insurers in Medicare Advantage programs.

- Increase transparency of cost and quality data.

- Full disclosure and transparency of payments and incentives to providers by drug or device makers that may lead to biased decision making.

- Overhaul of medical malpractice laws to lower costs while ensuring that injured patients receive fair compensation for their loss.

- Reform of long-term care services and support that shifts from institutionalization to care in the home and the community.

- Reform the tax code to empower consumers to spend their health care dollars wisely.

EVENT 2: EXPANSION OF THE STATE CHILDREN'S HEALTH INSURANCE PROGRAM (SCHIP)

The first legislative victory in health care reform came on February 4, 2009. This was the day President Obama signed into law the re-authorization of the SCHIP program. This bill (H.R.2)—passed by both the House and the Senate—increased SCHIP spending by $32.8 billion over the next 4 ½ years (2). The bill expanded coverage to over 4 million more children and added to the 6 million uninsured children from working families who are not poor enough to qualify for Medicaid. This bill will provide expanded coverage to 11 million children by 2013. This bill also provided dental benefits and parity for mental health benefits, and was funded by a 62-cent-per-pack increase in the federal cigarette tax.

EVENT 3: AMERICAN RECOVERY AND REINVESTMENT ACT (ARRA)

Following closely on the heels of SCHIP was the passing (although with strong Republican opposition) of the American Recovery and Reinvestment Act (ARRA) on February 17, 2009. This was a $789 billion stimulus bill that contained a package of spending increases and tax reliefs intended to spur an economic recovery and create jobs by putting money back in the pockets of consumers and companies. It was aimed at saving or creating 3.6 million jobs (3).

Interestingly, there were major health-related provisions in the ARRA bill that gave insight into what the president and Congress were considering for the health care reform bills that would follow. ARRA provided $111 billion in subsidies to extend COBRA insurance to newly unemployed workers. It also increased federal matching funds to help states maintain their Medicaid programs in the face of massive state budget shortfalls. Provisions were also included for Medicare payments to hospice, long term care hospitals, nursing facilities, hospitals, and Indian health provisions. The bill further included $19 billion as incentives for effective adoption of electronic technology designed to jump start physicians and hospitals into the Information Age. It started to standardize interoperability and the development of transparent processes, standards, and outcomes through a new Office of the National Coordinator for Health Information Technology (ONCHIT). The bill directed $1.1 billion to the Agency for Health Care Research and Quality (AHRQ) to help conduct evidence-based research to identify treatments, medications, radiologic imaging, procedures, and medical devices that are more effective than others in producing quality health care outcomes. Approximately $3 billion was put into the ARRA bill to encourage the health care system to refocus on prevention and wellness. It directed $500 million towards improving the primary care workforce in an attempt to build up the number of primary care physicians, physician assistants, and nurse practitioners who work in team-based primary care practices. Finally, the ARRA bill sustained and expanded the viability of the nation's CHCs (federally funded community health centers) that provide integrated and coordinated primary medical care, dental care, mental health care, pharmacy services, and associated social services to those in the community who struggle to get health care.

Taken collectively, these major health-related provisions in the ARRA stimulus bill delivered a first installment of presidential and congressional intent for a more accessible, efficient, evidence-based health care system that would be built on primary care and information technology and that would focus on wellness and prevention. The fourth and final event that helped shape health care reform is described below:

EVENT 4: WHITE HOUSE SUMMIT ON HEALTH CARE REFORM, MARCH 5, 2009

On March 5, 2009, President Barack Obama held a Health Care Reform Summit in the East Room of the White House. At this summit, approximately 250 key leaders in health care gathered from across our nation. They represented hospital organizations, physician groups, big business, small business, unions, consumer organizations, nursing organizations, health insurance companies, medical device manufacturers, pharmaceutical companies, and key leaders on the health care committees of the U.S. Senate and House of Representatives. I had the honor of participating in this summit. During this session, President Obama made it very clear to the assembled group that three things needed to happen in health care reform: 1) the status quo was unacceptable, 2) everyone must give a little bit for health care reform to move forward, and 3) we must do this, this year (4).

President Obama articulated that the costs of health care were bankrupting us, our states because of rising Medicaid costs, and our federal government due to rising Medicare costs and looming Medicare insolvency. These costs were affecting big business' ability to conduct business and the small business' ability to continue to provide health care insurance for their employees. He also acknowledged that the cost of health care was unaffordable to individual Americans. Premiums were increasing four times faster than wages and personal bankruptcies were happening every 30 seconds in America, leading to about 1.5 million personal bankruptcies per year (4). He made it very clear that the biggest economic threat to our country's fiscal health was health care; that cost control was not only a moral imperative, it was an absolute fiscal imperative for our country.

The second thing he included in health care reform goals was expansion of coverage. The president signaled this by signing into law the expansion of the State Children's Health Insurance Program (SCHIP) as his first bill. This expanded health care benefits to children and increased their coverage. He also expanded coverage in the ARRA stimulus bill to help states cover unemployed workers. He did not want the states to cut Medicaid benefits and he knew that states were struggling to balance their budgets during the downturn in the economy. The rates of the unemployed and uninsured were rising and this was something that health care reform must help correct.

The third thing that President Obama pointed to in his White House Summit was that America must invest in prevention, in a reform approach that guaranteed more people health care focused on wellness and prevention, and that this would in the long run absolutely save America money.

Figure 1. Ted Epperly, MD, Addressing President Obama at the White House Summit on Health Care Reform on March 5, 2009 (5)

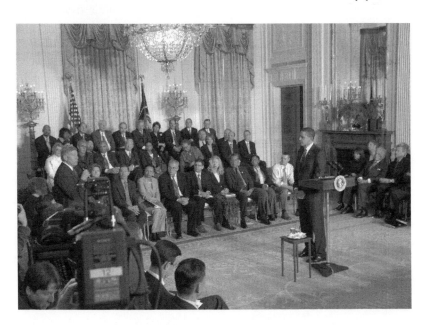

At the White House Summit it became clear that he wanted to start the transparent and open process from the bottom up by bringing the right people to the table quickly to work together for the best interests of our country to achieve health care reform. President Obama knew that this could not be a White House-administered proposal. He knew that the final health care reform bill must be a congressionally administered bill from both the House of Representatives and the Senate. Little did we all know at that time how big of an issue health care reform and its debate was to become. President Obama also signaled a sense of urgency. He recognized that we must do this within a year so that politics as usual in Washington, special interest groups, and the failures of the past could not again overwhelm the efforts and produce a stalemate that would mean a continuation and worsening of the present problem.

So, to summarize, the Baucus Call to Action White Paper, the expansion of the State Children's Health Insurance Program (SCHIP), the American Recovery and Reinvestment Act (ARRA), and President Obama's White House Health Reform Summit became the foundation on which the House and Senate built their health care reform bills. This foundation was the base on which the three committees of the House (Ways and Means, Energy and Commerce, Education and Labor) and the two committees of the Senate (Senate Finance and Senate Health, Education, Labor, and Pensions) started to construct their bills. At this stage of health care reform there was much focused work around health care policies. Good ideas from both Republicans and Democrats were being weighed and evaluated to construct these bills. At this juncture, health care reform was not a Democratic or Republican issue, but an American issue. The thinking at this time was that we did not need to burn down our health care system and create a new one, nor did we need to copy one from another country. The assumption of the House and the Senate was that we would build on top of what was good about our existing health care system and add layers to it that would help improve, reform, and simplify it for the good of our country. Unfolding from the events described, the health care reform measures tackled in the three committees in the House of Representatives and the two committees in the Senate can be organized into six major pillars of health care reform. Figure 2 below depicts my view of these six pillars built on top of our existing health care system.

Figure 2. The Six Pillars of Health Care Reform

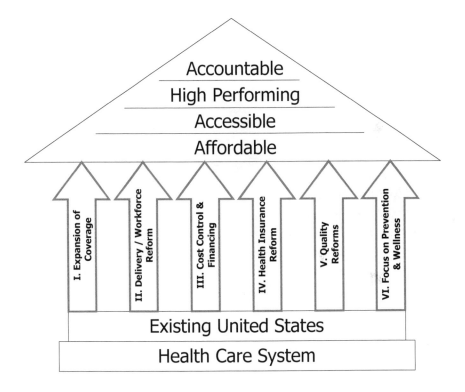

Figure 3 provides some basic information about House Bill H.R.3962, the Affordable Health Care for America Act and Senate Bill H.R.3590, the Patient Protection and Affordable Care Act. The information in the following sections is derived from two excellent publications, one from the Henry Kaiser Family Foundation (6) and the other from The Commonwealth Fund (7).

Figure 3. Final Health Care Reform Bills—A Side-by-Side Comparison

	House Bill (H.R.3962)	Senate Bill (H.R.3590)
Bill Name	Affordable Health Care for America Act	Patient Protection and Affordable Care Act
Announced	October 29, 2009	November 18, 2009
Manager's Amendment	–	December 19, 2009
Passed	November 7, 2009	December 24, 2009
Vote	220–215	60–39
Number of Pages	1990	906

The "six pillars" offered a framework for the construction of a reformed health care system. This structure was to be created by two different teams of builders (the House and Senate), sometimes working from a common plan and sometimes from noticeably different views of what the final result would be. Let's take an aerial view of this process, flying high enough to see the major details without getting bogged down too much by the smallest details on the capitals of each pillar.

PILLAR ONE: EXPANSION OF COVERAGE

Percent of Americans Covered

The health care reform bills that were passed by the Senate (the Patient Protection and Affordable Health Care Act) and the House (the Affordable Health Care for America Act) expanded coverage to the uninsured and also helped protect the underinsured. On the Senate side this expansion was to approximately 94 percent of all

Americans. It was about 97 percent in the House bill. Without this expanded coverage the number of uninsured would increase to 54 million people by 2019 (8).

Individual Mandate

Provisions in both the Senate and the House bills required that U.S. citizens and legal residents have individual mandated health insurance. Penalty for not following the mandate in the House bill was 2.5 percent of income and in the Senate bill the greater of either $750 or 2 percent of income.

Employer Mandate

On the House side, employers must pay 72.5 percent of the premium for single coverage and 65 percent of the premium for families (or 8 percent of payroll). Businesses with less than $500,000 on payroll were exempt, and payrolls up to $750,000 would require a reduced contribution. In the Senate bill there was no requirement for employers to offer health insurance. However, employers with more than 50 employees that do not offer coverage would be assessed a fee of $750 for every employee. Employers with less than 50 employees would have been exempt from these penalties.

Medicaid Expansion

Both the House and the Senate would have increased expansion of Medicaid programs. The House bill would have expanded Medicaid coverage to all Americans with incomes below 150 percent of the federal poverty level. In the Senate bill Medicaid would have been expanded to everyone below 133 percent of the federal poverty level.

Health Insurance Exchanges

Both bills also called for the creation of health insurance exchanges to give people more health insurance options from a marketplace with multiple plans. The Senate bill created a state-based American

Health Benefit Exchange through which individuals could purchase coverage, while the House bill created a Federal Health Insurance Exchange through which individuals and smaller employers could purchase health coverage.

Individual Subsidies

To help people pay for mandated plans, individuals and families who earn up to 400 percent of the federal poverty level under the Senate bill would have received tax credits. The House bill included the same provision.

Public Plan Option

Another federal program, offered through the Health Insurance Exchange, was termed the Public Plan Option, which would have expanded coverage choices and drove health insurance reform through direct competition with private health insurance companies. This plan option would have had the same requirements as private plans regarding benefit levels, provider networks, consumer protections, and cost sharing. In the House bill this would have been set up and run by the secretary of Health and Human Services. In the House bill the HHS secretary would have negotiated provider rates which would not be lower than Medicare rates and not higher than the average rates paid by other qualified private insurers. In the Senate bill there was no provision for a Public Plan Option, but instead it allowed private insurers to offer national insurance policies to Americans across state lines.

Abortion Coverage

Clear firewalls were placed into the bills on both the Senate and the House side to prevent funding abortions outside of those that protect the life of the mother or for rape or incest.

Benefit Package

The basic benefit package of both the Senate and House health care reform bills set the basic minimum that all health insurance plans would provide in order to be included in the health insurance exchanges. In the Senate bill the secretary of Health and Human Services defined and annually updated the benefit package through a transparent and public process. In the House version of the bill, a Health Benefits Advisory Council, chaired by the surgeon general, made recommendations on services to be covered.

Benefit Categories

In both bills there were provisions for four benefit categories. On the Senate side these constituted the bronze, silver, gold, and platinum plans. They differed by the percentage of the benefit costs covered by the plans: bronze was 60 percent; silver, 70 percent; gold, 80 percent; and platinum, 90 percent. The Senate bill also covered a catastrophic plan. On the House side the four benefit categories were the basic plan (70 percent coverage), the enhanced plan (85 percent coverage), the premium plan (95 percent coverage), and the premium plus plan (95 percent coverage plus additional benefits including oral health and vision care).

PILLAR TWO: DELIVERY/WORKFORCE REFORM

The second pillar of reform is delivery and workforce. It is one thing to expand coverage to approximately 94 percent to 97 percent of the people in this country. However, if you do not have the right type of workforce of physicians to care for those people, you have only compounded the problem with issues of access, timeliness of care, and seeing the right types of physicians, in the right places, for the right reasons, at the right time. This is exactly the problem that happened in the state of Massachusetts. In 2006, the state of Massachusetts gave 97.6 percent of health insurance coverage to all of the commonwealth's citizens. However, the state lacked the right type of primary care physician workforce. This led to longer waiting times, up to 100-day waits for certain physicians (9). Emergency room utilization increased dramatically and drove up the cost of health care. This is why the delivery and workforce side of health care reform is so critical. You cannot give expanded coverage without expanded workforce of the right type of physicians. This was the message I delivered to President Obama at the White House Summit on Health Care Reform. Unfortunately, as was pointed out in earlier chapters, America has a very distorted and broken physician workforce.

Advisory Committee on Health Workforce

The first large step for the United States in putting together a workforce strategy was forming an Advisory Committee on Health Workforce. We lack an overarching strategy for the numbers or types of physicians we train in this country. We have left this totally open to free-market forces. In our health care system we do not pay to keep people healthy, we pay to treat people after they become unhealthy. Therefore, our workforce has been attracted to subspecialties and medicine that focus on procedures and imaging, as these are better paid for than basic primary care. The creation of a Workforce Advisory Committee in the Senate bill or an Advisory Committee on Health Workforce in the House bill was thus critical. We obviously need multiple types of physician groups. Our problem is that we need a better balance. We must refocus on developing more physicians that can go out into the inner-city urban, suburban, and rural areas and provide outstanding community-based health care. We need to create the right types of physicians who can fix the problem.

Primary Care and General Surgeon Payment

If we want more primary care physicians and general surgeons emerging from America's medical schools, we must fix the system of how physicians are paid. We must focus on the front end of medicine and pay more for health, wellness, prevention, and chronic disease management, and less for high-end procedures and imaging for people who become ill from lack of early care.

This is a re-aiming at the target of keeping people healthy and in less need of medical services. Steps in this direction were taken in the reform bills with the Senate increasing primary care payment by 10 percent for five years. In the House bill this payment was a permanent 5 percent increase that went to 10 percent in rural and underserved areas.

Graduate Medical Education (GME) Redistribution

Graduate medical education (GME), or residency, refers to the training after a physician's graduation from medical school until he or she is ready for full medical practice without supervision. Physicians in this residency training are called interns in the first year and residents in the remaining years of training. There are 24 different specialties of medicine (e.g., family medicine, pediatrics, internal medicine, general surgery, radiology, etc.), and each specialty has a GME program, which varies in length from three years in primary care areas to seven years in the subspecialty of neurosurgery. A provision of the bills moved unused residency slots from subspecialty areas into training primary care and general surgical physicians. This would be prioritized, at least on the Senate side, to states with the lowest resident physician to population ratios. The bills also worked to achieve more training flexibility outside of large teaching hospitals and academic medical centers by focusing on community and outpatient clinic settings. It is in these community-based settings where health, wellness, chronic disease management, and prevention often happen and is focused on team-based education where physicians work with nurses, nurse practitioners, physician assistants, nutritionists, social workers, psychologists, pharmacists, and others critical to health care teams. The Senate also tried to ensure the availability of residency programs in rural and underserved areas. This was a bold and exciting step to train and develop a workforce differently than the model that has been used for the last hundred years.

Teaching Health Centers

One exciting new concept introduced in both the Senate and House bill was the concept of teaching health centers (THC). These are hybrids of residency programs, primarily in family medicine but also in internal medicine and pediatrics, with community health centers (CHC, federally designated clinics made up of primary care physicians). CHCs also provide much-needed mental health care, dental health care, and pharmacy services, and act as "safety net" providers to communities, providing much needed primary care services to the poor, the elderly, and the uninsured. There are approximately 1,250 CHCs across America serving approximately 20 million patients (10). These new teaching health centers would fuse together in new ways these education programs with the community health centers, thereby creating new hybrids of education and service.

Scholarship and Loan Repayment

For primary care physicians and general surgeons, there was an increase in National Health Service Corps funding (NHSC) to provide scholarships, on the front end, as well as loan repayment for medical school debt on the back end if these physicians go into rural and underserved areas.

Support Primary Care Training: Title VII–Section 747, Family Medicine Training

Both bills contained provisions to support primary care training and capacity through Title VII. Section 747 of the Public Health Service Act is specific to training in family medicine. This would continue grants for the training of family physicians both in medical schools, departments of family medicine, and family medicine residencies. This is the only funding mechanism in the entire federal budget at this time to try and support this critical family medicine training pipeline. Of the $9 billion spent per year on graduate medical education (GME), only about $54 million (0.5 percent) goes into Title

VII–Section 747 to support the infrastructure for family medicine training (11).

Mental, Behavioral, and Oral Health Training

Both bills worked toward developing interdisciplinary training models to amplify mental and behavioral health training, as well as oral health training. Much of the training in the United States healthcare system is done in silos. Each specialty in medicine often does not train with other specialties in medicine and rarely is there any interprofessional training between physicians, nurses, dentists, psychologists, or social workers. These provisions would call for different training models that would start to integrate the system better. This model focused these important disciplines into community-based clinics and away from hospitals so that these services could be accessed by patients and people where they most need them.

Expand Nursing Education

Both the Senate and the House bills included provisions to address the anticipated shortage of nurses. Legislation in the bills was written to help not only increase the training but also the retention of nurses by providing loan repayments and retention grants.

Nurse-Managed Health Clinics

The utilization of nurse practitioners (NP) and physician assistants (PA) will be very important to help alleviate the physician workforce crisis. There were provisions in both the Senate and House bills to increase nurse-managed clinics in which appropriately trained nurse practitioners would care for patients within the scope of their practice, their license, and their abilities. These nurse-managed health clinics would be done without physician supervision or oversight in states that allow independent nurse practitioner practice.

Patient-Centered Medical Homes/Integrated Teams

Both bills contained provisions for integrated training that bring together primary care, behavioral care, and chronic disease management in the concept of the patient-centered medical home (PCMH). A PCMH is a location (a primary care practice) and a system of care that integrates continuity of care over time with a team-based approach to the entirety of the patient's health care needs. It is a one-stop location that is timely, accessible, and focuses on not only acute and chronic problems but, just as importantly, on wellness, prevention, and behavioral modification that leads to health. More about PCMHs later.

Community Health Centers (CHCs)/School-Based Health Centers (SBHCs)

Both bills would have increased funding for community health centers and school-based health centers (SBHC). In the House version of the bill there would be $12 billion increase in funding over five years to help support and expand CHCs and SBHCs. Since the expanded medical team at a CHC is made up heavily of family physicians and other primary care physicians, it could easily become a PCMH. The location and process of care with integration, coordination, continuity, and comprehensiveness fit perfectly into what CHCs can provide to their patients and communities.

Public Health and Disaster Preparedness

We must start thinking more about the health of our communities as a whole and not just the individuals in them, focusing on air and water quality, immunization rates, and control and prevention of infectious diseases. Public health around obesity, increased exercise, and better nutrition must also be priorities. The House bill provided grants to each state's health departments for such activities and public health infrastructure development. The Senate bill focused more on disaster preparedness and the establishment of a commissioned regular corps and a ready reserve corps in times of a national emergency.

Trauma Care

The House bill proposed to create a new trauma center program in urban areas, especially around violent crimes. This bill would help further develop the infrastructure of emergency departments and trauma centers. It would also create the Emergency Care Coordination Center in the Department of Health and Human Services. The Senate had no similar provision.

American Indians

Both the Senate and House bills reauthorized and amended the Indian Health Care Improvement Act. This is important as our nation continues to provide timely and high-quality care to the American Indian population.

PILLAR THREE: COST CONTROL AND FINANCING

As has been noted earlier, the projected growth of health care spending in the gross domestic product goes from 17 percent today to 25 percent in the year 2025, and to 50 percent in the year 2082 (12). Both the Senate and House bills tried to reduce the exploding cost of health care primarily by looking for cost reductions in Medicare and Medicaid, and in administrative simplification, waste fraud and abuse reduction, and prescription drug utilization.

Congressional Budget Office (CBO) Estimated Cost and Deficit Reduction

The Congressional Budget Office estimated the cost of this reform to be approximately $871 billion over 10 years on the Senate side of the reform bill, and a little over $1 trillion over 10 years in the House bill. Our current health care system costs $2.6 trillion a year.

Therefore, an increase of $871 billion (Senate) to $1,052 billion (House) over 10 years or $87 billion to $105 billion per year is only a 3.3 percent to 4.0 percent increase per year, much slower than the current health care inflation rate. It would bring us long term, meaningful reform, an idea often lost in the rhetoric and the politics. This is a bargain and will result in a deficit reduction of $132 billion over 10 years on the Senate side, and $104 billion over 10 years on the House side. Why would we not invest now to start to save later? It should be noted that within these numbers are $426 billion (House) to $438 billion (Senate) savings in Medicare and Medicaid over these 10 years.

Administrative Simplification

Both bills called for long overdue health insurance forms simplification. The Senate bill called for a single set of operating rules for eligibility verification and claims status, electronic funds transfers, and health care payments. The House bill called for similar standards of electronic transactions and for timely and transparent claims.

Eliminate Waste, Fraud, and Abuse

Both bills called for reducing and ideally eliminating waste, fraud, and abuse in all public programs. Fortunately, there is not as much purposeful fraud and abuse as there is just mindless waste and inefficiency. This again was at the core of Baucus' statement that one-third of health care spending is unneeded or wasted. That is $800 billion per year!

Prescription Drugs

The House bill called for enhanced competition between brand name and generic drug manufacturers to stop agreements that limit, delay, or prevent competition. The Senate bill authorized new "biologic" drugs 12 years of exclusive use before generic drugs can be developed, to allow these pharmaceutical companies sufficient time to recoup research, development, and marketing costs before competition with generics starts.

New Models of Care: Patient-Centered Medical Home (PCMH) and Accountable Care Organizations (ACOs)

Patient-Centered Medical Home (PCMH)

An example of how we can better integrate and coordinate health care and save cost at the practice level is through patient-centered medical homes (PCMH), based on patients having a personal trusted primary care physician. A well-trained primary care physician can take care of multiple problems at the same time in one patient visit and orchestrate what needs to be done. The primary care physician can look into the patient's eyes who is suffering from diabetes, heart failure, and depression and say, "Mrs. Smith, we need to have these two tests done, but we do not need these other five tests done because they are unnecessary at this time to focus on your best health." Without this personal primary physician relationship in the PCMH, Mrs. Smith may be loose in the system, receiving high-cost, fragmented care from a disparate number of providers from either the emergency room or different subspecialists, in which the care is not integrated into one comprehensive plan for the good of the patient. In this case she may receive not only those other five tests but perhaps 10 other tests leading to more cost, confusion, and potential harm to the patient. Many of the cost-saving reductions in both Medicare and Medicaid can happen by having such a system as the PCMH; one that delivers appropriate levels of care, rendered by the right physician, at the right place, at the right time, and for the right reasons.

Accountable Care Organizations (ACOs)

Another example of a health care delivery model at the larger systems level is the Accountable Care Organizations (ACOs). These are vertically integrated entities that deliver health care through teams of providers from initial contact with primary care physicians and emergency room physicians, all the way through subspecialty utilization, hospital care, and rehabilitative care for the patient as needed. An episode of hospital care would span from three days before an event, such as a hospital admission, to 30 days after the patient has been discharged. This episode of illness, injury, or care will then be paid for in a bundled amount, distributed among all the providers involved in care. This moves away from each provider charging a fee for each individual service but rather the ACO charging one global fee. This model will be incentivized to provide high-quality, efficient care that maximizes integration, coordination, and teamwork and lowers cost.

The integration of primary care physicians and their expanded teams in the PCMH model will fit nicely into the larger, vertically integrated ACOs. Patients are cared for in a timely, accessible way by their primary care physicians. If the patient needs further care, the patient can then be appropriately routed into an ACO in which efficiency, integration, coordination, and accountability can occur.

The PCMH and the ACO are examples of model reform on the delivery side that would impact the cost of health care. They would avoid redundancy, duplication, and fragmentation, which is what is responsible for the $800 billion a year that Senator Baucus said was lost in the health care system through waste (1).

PILLAR FOUR: HEALTH INSURANCE REFORM

One of the most important areas of reform tackled by Congress was health insurance. The balance of power has shifted away from patients, and families, and businesses into the hands of the insurance companies that have held far too much power to determine who is covered, for what conditions, and at what cost. When insurance premiums are rising four times faster than wages, this becomes a problem to individuals, families, and businesses. Both the House and Senate health care reform bills contained measures that would do the following (13):

1. Eliminate discrimination for preexisting conditions.

2. Guarantee insurance renewal.

3. Allow no lifetime caps on total coverage.

4. Eliminate exorbitant, out-of-pocket expenses, deductibles, or co-pays.

5. Eliminate dropping of coverage for those who become seriously ill.

6. Require insurance companies to cover regular checkups and preventive exams.

7. Forbid gender discrimination in assigning rates.

8. Extend coverage for young adults as part of family coverage through the age of 26.

These reforms would guarantee that the insurance companies must play by new rules that are fairly and equitably applied.

Guaranteed Issue and Rating Rules

Both bills contained requirements for guaranteed issue and renewability. Rating variation could only be based on age, geographic area, family size, and tobacco use.

Temporary High-Risk Pool

Both bills established temporary national high-risk pools to provide health insurance coverage to individuals, spouses, and dependents with preexisting medical conditions that were uninsured for at least six months. These provisions were put in place to act as a bridge until health insurance exchanges could be developed in each state to ensure that high-risk patients with complex medical problems would be afforded health insurance coverage.

Medical Loss Ratio and Premium Rate Reviews

Both bills required health plans to report the percentage of premium dollars spent on clinical services, quality, and other costs. The bills required at least 85 percent of premium dollars to be spent on clinical services (i.e., medical loss ratio). This lowered to 80 percent in the Senate bill for plans in the individual and small group market.

Administrative Simplification

Both bills called for standards for administrative and financial transaction simplification.

Dependent Coverage

Both bills called for expanded dependent children coverage—to age 26 in the Senate bill and age 27 in the House bill.

Insurance Market Rules

Both bills prohibited placing lifetime limits on coverage, exclusions for preexisting conditions unless cases of fraud. The Senate bill also required all new policies to comply with one of the four benefit categories and to limit deductibles to $2,000 for individuals and $4,000 for families. The Senate bill also penalized employers that have a waiting period of greater than 60 days for employees to receive coverage. The House bill also called for extension of COBRA coverage until the health insurance exchanges were established.

Consumer Protections

Both bills developed uniform marketing standards and standards for information on benefits and coverage.

Selling Insurance Across State Lines

Both bills allowed states to form health care choice compacts that enabled insurers to sell policies across state lines in any state participating in the compact. The result would be increased competition for insurance products based on quality and cost.

Anti-Trust Exemption

The House bill called for removal of anti-trust exemptions for both health and medical malpractice insurers. Before this, both of these entities could participate in discussions about setting prices on health insurance and medical liability prices at the expense of both doctors and patients. The Senate bill had no similar provision.

PILLAR FIVE: QUALITY REFORMS

As has been discussed earlier in the book, America has the highest cost health care system in the world, weighing in at $2.6 trillion spent per year, roughly $8,500 each for every man, woman, and child in our country. At the same time, the measures of our quality rank us mediocre at best.

One of the overarching goals of health care reform is to get our nation to a high-value, high-quality system. The best definition I have ever heard of value is that value equals quality divided by cost. Therefore, anything that drives up quality while holding cost stable will be a value to health care. Conversely, if quality can be held stable and cost reduced, then that also increases the value of health care. The most impressive increases in value are when quality goes up and cost goes down. This is the main focus of quality reform. It increases the value of health care for our country and our nation as a whole.

National Quality Strategy

Both the Senate and House bills addressed quality issues including development of a National Center for Quality Improvement. America has a fragmented health care system made up of many moving parts that for the most part are unregulated, uncontrolled, unchecked, uncoordinated, and unaccountable. An overarching quality strategy was proposed to help connect these disparate parts into a better-functioning whole.

Quality Measures

Both bills created processes and priorities for performance improvement and quality measures. These priorities and measures would be developed by multiple stakeholders, and would be used in both reporting and payment for federal programs such as Medicare, Medicaid, and Tricare (the military insurance program).

Medical Homes

The Senate bill created a Medicaid state plan that would allow patients with at least two chronic conditions, one condition and risk of developing another, or at least one serious condition and persistent mental health condition, to designate a provider/practice as their "health home." The bills spoke again to the creation of these "medical homes" or "health homes" in both the Medicaid and Medicare programs as a way to coordinate and integrate care.

Bundled Payments

Both bills called for pilot programs (Senate) or a plan (House) to develop and evaluate bundled, composite payments in both Medicare and Medicaid programs for acute, inpatient hospital services, physician services, outpatient hospital services, and post-acute care services. This "episode of care" would begin roughly three days prior to a hospitalization and spans 30 days following discharge.

Community-Based Collaborative Care Network Program

An innovative idea was the establishment of what has been called a Community-Based Collaborative Care Network Program. This was present in both the Senate and House bills and supported a consortium of health care providers to coordinate and integrate health care services for low-income, uninsured, and underinsured populations. The outcomes as stated in the House bill would be to reduce emergency room utilization and hospital admissions.

Independence at Home Demonstration Programs

A high-functioning health care system of the future will start to care more for patients in the community setting and in their home setting than in hospitals. To move in this direction, incentives were provided in both the Senate and House bills for home demonstration programs. These programs would take high-need Medicare patients and link them to needed primary care services that would be coordinated with other teams of health professionals such as home health agencies. This would be ongoing, proactive care to keep people healthy and maximally functional in the home setting, thus decreasing the need for hospital admissions, ER visits, and hospital readmissions.

Hospital-Based Purchasing

Since hospitals cannot totally go away, programs would be implemented in the Senate bill that would look at different ways in which to pay hospitals based on performance and on achieving quality measures. This was only in the Senate bill and this provision was not in the House bill.

Geographic Variations

In the House version of the health care reform bill there was a requirement for the Institute of Medicine to conduct a study on geographic variation and adjustment factors for Medicare patients. The results were to be reported to the secretary of Health and Human Services and would result in revised geographic adjustment factors. Again, this was in an attempt to understand why there should be such regionally disparate outcomes in terms of quality and cost.

Health Care Disparities

Both bills contained legislation that would require enhanced collection and reporting of data on variations in quality and cost that occur along racial, ethnic, gender, and disability lines, as well as variations in underserved, rural, and frontier populations. Again, the focus would be to increase value by driving up quality and lowering cost.

Comparative Effectiveness Research

Both the Senate and the House bills developed language around use of research at the point of care between physicians and their patients in order to drive higher quality and to lower cost. This research data would be evidence-based and would help support the patient and his or her physician in making the most appropriate choices. This received a lot of heat, primarily around the issue of whether or not the data would be used to ration or deny care. In the Senate bill a non-profit Patient-Centered Outcomes Research Institute would be created to provide this information on clinical effectiveness of medical treatments. On the House side this center would be created within the Agency for Health Care Research and Quality (AHRQ) of Health and Human Services. In neither bill would mandates or guidelines be developed to deny coverage or ration care.

Financial Disclosure

An area introduced in both bills would call for full financial disclosures to occur and be transparent to the public between physicians, hospitals, pharmaceutical companies, pharmacists, medical device manufacturers, biologicals, and other health-related entities. This was included to help ensure that bias was not being applied by any of these groups in regards to how health care was being decided on or performed.

PILLAR SIX: FOCUS ON PREVENTION AND WELLNESS

Our nation's health care system has been built around reactive, high cost, illness and injury medicine, not around prevention, wellness, and excellent chronic disease management. We must get to a more proactive, front end of health care and start to decrease the high-cost, reactive, procedure-laden, back-end health care system we have.

National Strategy

Provisions were put in the Senate bill to establish the National Prevention

Health Promotion and Public Health Council to oversee development of a strategy to improve the nation's health. This strategy would help the nation coordinate and align education, payments, patient incentives, and other activities to drive a health care system instead of a sick care system. The House bill contained a provision for the development of a national strategy to improve the nation's health through task forces that would develop, update, and disseminate evidence-based recommendations on the use of clinical and community prevention services.

Grants Program

Within this strategy was the development of a nationalized grant program to support the delivery of evidence-based services and community-based prevention and wellness programs aimed at strengthening the community's health and decreasing disparities and poor health care outcomes. In addition, the House bill called for training community health workers to promote positive health behaviors, especially in medically underserved areas. The House bill also provided grants for obesity prevention among children and families.

Prevention Services Coverage

Another way to improve prevention is to fully cover the cost of evidence-based preventive services. This was done for both Medicare and Medicaid patients in these bills. The Senate bill also required qualified health plans to provide coverage without cost sharing for preventive services. The United States Preventative Services Task Force (USPSTF) data would be utilized for these decisions based on a rating system concerning recommendations for immunizations and preventive services for infants, children, adolescents, and women. The House bill contained a similar provision.

Health Risk Assessment

The Senate bill contained a provision to allow Medicare beneficiaries a one-time "Welcome to Medicare" visit that would develop a health risk assessment and a personalized prevention plan for the new patient. There were also provisions to Medicare and Medicaid beneficiaries to complete behavior modification programs.

Wellness Programs

Another effective way to get patients as groups involved with their own health care would be to provide incentives for employers to provide wellness programs. Larger groups of people can motivate each other to increase the health of the employees as a whole, resulting in a healthier workforce. It would also decrease the costs of health care expended as these people focus on their health. The Senate bill provided grants for up to five years to small employers to establish these programs. On the House side grants were for up to three years and covered up to 50 percent of costs incurred for these programs. There was also coverage for technical assistance to employers in how to best do this. Employers would provide rewards (e.g., premium discounts, waivers of cost sharing) to their employees for participation and improvement.

Nutrition Information

There were provisions in both the House and Senate bills to provide nutritional information to the public through chain restaurants and their menus, and for food sold from vending machines. This was an effort to engage patients with education and their awareness of the calorie counts and trans fats in these items.

Preventive Medicine and Public Health Education

The Senate bill contained a provision for medical physicians in training (residents) to be provided with more training in preventive care and public health. This is being done in the primary care programs now. However, this should extend to all residency programs so all physicians are more aware and in tune with these principles to help create a proactive educational environment around health care and not sick care.

OTHER AREAS OF REFORM

There are three other parts of the health care reform bills that do not fall into these large six pillars that need to be mentioned. These are items around liability reform, long-term nursing home care, and prescription drug coverage.

Liability Reform

The physician community and many others were disappointed that there was not more in these health care reform bills around liability reform. The practice of defensive medicine is known to increase the cost of health care because physicians over-order lab tests, radiologic imaging, and consultation with others, to ensure that they're not missing something. They also tend to over-diagnose and over-prescribe medications for the same reason. Ordering more tests and doing more procedures does not equate to better health outcomes. In fact more testing, medications, procedures, and consultations can lead to more mistakes, errors in communication, and issues of clinical irrelevance that are discovered and then lead to another round of testing, procedures, and consultation. Too much health care can be toxic to health. Too much health care can definitely lower quality of health care outcomes. All of this has a direct cost on health care as well as on its quality. In a study published in 2007 the total impact of the current tort system on medical expenses and the cost of defensive medicine is approximately $124 billion per year (14). Therefore, liability reform in the health care reform bills is paramount in decreasing the cost of the health care system while increasing quality outcomes.

Congress did not enact larger reform principles around medical liability because of the power of the trial lawyer lobby and the fact that many Congressmen are lawyers. It is hard to truly appreciate why this very important provision was not dealt with more boldly. There were provisions in both the Senate and the House bills around medical malpractice. The Senate bill provided awards to states for five-year demonstration grants to develop, implement, and evaluate alternatives to current tort litigations. On the House side these were incentive payments to states that develop alternative medical liability laws that provide prompt and fair resolution of disputes, disclosure of medical errors, and affordable liability insurance. It is a sad statement that many health care providers stop the provision of certain needed health care services (e.g., obstetrical care) in their community because they cannot afford the liability insurance. This must be fixed with future laws.

Long-Term Care

America is aging and there will soon be a doubling of our Medicare population from 40 to 80 million people, so proactive steps need to be taken regarding long-term care provisions and planning. If possible, it is best for both the patient and the family if the elderly can be cared for in their home and in their community by people they know and trust. Recognizing that is not always the case nor is it always possible, a balance of reform efforts need to be attempted to ensure high-quality and low-cost care occur in these settings.

CLASS Act

In both the Senate and the House bills were provisions for the CLASS program, which stands for Community Living Assistance Services and Supports. The language of both bills included the establishment of a national, voluntary insurance program to purchase these types of services and support.

Home Care Options

Along these lines in the Senate bill were provisions for Medicaid reform that would provide states with new options for offering home and community-based services under a state's Medicaid plan. These plans would provide for attendants, supports, and services to individuals with disabilities who require institutional level care. Additionally, the Senate bill contained provisions for federal matching programs to eligible states to increase the proportion of noninstitutionally bound long-term care services. All of these taken together will help states, families, and individuals focus more on ambulatory, community-based care rather than long-term institutionally based care.

Skilled Nursing Facility Requirements

Both the Senate and House bills contained provisions for transparency of reporting of data regarding ownership, expenditures, and accountability requirements for skilled nursing facilities under Medicare and nursing facilities under Medicaid.

The Core Competencies for Personal and Home Care Aides

The House bill also had a three-year demonstration project in four states to measure the effectiveness of recommended core competencies for all personal and home care aides.

Prescription Medication Coverage/"Donut Hole" Reduction

Prescription medication coverage is another long overdue health care reform. This reform focuses on eliminating the donut hole of medication coverage for Medicare patients on Part D Medicare. The way Part D coverage works is that a certain amount of Medicare coverage is provided until a threshold is reached and then there is no coverage until an upper maximum amount is reached, at which point Medicare coverage will then reoccur. This so-called donut hole is a gap in coverage and affects many Medicare aged patients. Language In both the Senate and House reform bills would increase Medicare Part D coverage and start to close this gap. Both bills closed the size of the donut hole and narrow the gap by $500 after health care reform is passed. On the House side the same gap elimination occurred by $500 initially, but went further to eliminate the Medicare Part D coverage gap (donut hole) totally by 2019.

Brand-Name Medication Cost Reduction

There were also provisions in both the House and Senate bills for a 50 percent discount on brand-name prescriptions covered under Medicare Part D for patients who are in the coverage gap.

The Senate and House bills together totaled nearly 3,000 pages of legislation to bring about sweeping health care reform. Figure 4 below outlines some of the major similarities between the two bills.

Figure 4. Major Similarities Between the House and Senate Bills

1. Coverage	• Expand Coverage • Individual Mandate • Premium and Cost-Sharing Subsidies • Medicaid/SCHIP Expansion
2. Delivery/Workforce Reform	• Advisory Committee on Workforce • Increase Payment for Primary Care and General Surgeons • Graduate Medical Education Redistribution • Expand Nursing Education
3. Cost Reform/Financing of Health Care	• Medicare and Medicaid Cost Savings/Center for Payment Innovation • Administrative Simplification • Eliminate Medicare/Medicaid Waste, Fraud, and Abuse
4. Health Insurance	• Insurance Market Regulation • Standard Benefit Packages
5. Quality Reforms	• National Quality Improvement Strategy • Comparative Effectiveness Research Center
6. Prevention and Wellness	• Create and Expand Prevention and Wellness Programs
7. Liability Reform	• Both with Minimal Reform; State Based
8. Long-Term Care	• Agree on Reform Changes Needed
9. Prescription Medication Coverage	• Agree on Most Changes

Figure 5 below outlines the major differences between the Senate bill and the House bill.

Figure 5. Major Differences Between the Bills

	Senate Bill (H.R. 3590)	House Bill (H.R. 3962)
1. Coverage		
• Percent Covered	94%	97%
• Employer Mandate	No	Yes
• Health Insurance Exchange	State	Federal
• Public Plan Option	No	Yes
2. Delivery Workforce Reform		
• Trauma Care	No	Yes
3. Cost Reform/Financing of Health Care		
• CBO Estimated Cost	$871 billion over 10 years	$1,052 billion over 10 years
• CBO Estimated Deficit Reduction	$132 billion over 10 years	$104 billion over 10 years
• Sources of Revenue	Excise tax on high-cost health plans	Increase taxation on high incomes
• Sustainable Growth Rate (SGR) Fix	No	Yes
• Independent Medicare Advisory Board	Yes	No
4. Health Insurance Reform		
• Remove Health Insurance Anti-Trust Exemption	No	Yes
5. Quality Reforms		
• Geographic Variation Differences	No	Yes
6. Prevention and Wellness		
• Welcome to Medicare Visit	Yes	No
7. Prescription Medication Coverage		
• Medicare Part D Gap Reduction	Partial	Total over time

With these major provisions of the bills in mind, let's now move onto our next chapter to see what happened to these health care reform efforts and bills.

Chapter 9

THE AFFORDABLE CARE ACT

As the year 2009 came to a close, America saw the passage of the House bill on November 7, 2009, and the Senate bill on Christmas Eve of 2009. All that was needed was to have a conference committee between the House and the Senate that would knit the two bills into one common final bill. This was historic—this would be the largest bill on health care reform since the passage of Medicare and Medicaid in 1965. As the year 2009 quietly slipped away and a new decade began, the two political parties and the American people's increasing uneasiness fomented the rancorous debate over health care reform. Continuous messaging from the Republican Party and right-wing media framed health care reform as bad for America. They portrayed a government takeover, loss of Medicare, the government getting between you and your physician, massive costs, and a piling up of the national deficit.

This played out, ironically, on the national stage in the most unlikely state of Massachusetts. Massachusetts to this point in time had been the bluest of the blue states. It had been considered the Democratic stronghold of America. It was the state in which progressive health care reform had been adopted in 2006. By 2009, 97.6 percent of its citizens had health care coverage. It was the state in which Senator Ted Kennedy, the champion of health care reform, had been the senior senator for 45 years. This was the state in which Ted Kennedy had hoped one day to see a better health care system for America become a reality.

But that all ended on January 19, 2010. That was the day that

Republican State Senator Scott Brown was elected in Massachusetts as the 41st vote to stop health care reform. Scott Brown, one of only five Republicans among the 40 state senators in Massachusetts, had just won a victory to become Massachusetts' newest United States Senator and shocked the nation! This was supposed to be an easy victory for Democrats. This was supposed to be a slam dunk to continue the Senate Democratic majority in the United States Senate. This was supposed to be a fait accompli to continue the momentum for health care reform for our country. But that is not what happened. Brown's position on health care was that he would give the Republicans the power to block what Brown called the "trillion-dollar health care bill that is being forced on the American people, one that will raise taxes, hurt Medicare, destroy jobs and run our nation deeper into debt." (1) Even though there was a three to one ratio of registered Democrats to registered Republicans in Massachusetts, almost half of the citizenry is Independent. Scott Brown won the majority of the Independents' votes, winning the race with a five-point margin.

This effectively killed health care reform as we knew it because the supermajority of 60 votes needed in the United States Senate no longer existed. Upon exit polling, the citizens of Massachusetts stated that they liked their state health care system but were growing unsettled by its rising cost and problems with access. What bothered them even more was the process they saw going on in Washington. The independent voters in Massachusetts who were likely to vote rose up and basically said, "We're sick of the politics as usual, we're tired of the political wrangling in Washington over health care reform, we have our system in place in Massachusetts, and so we're going to vote our conscience for the best candidate." (1) Scott Brown ran a campaign similar to Barack Obama's campaign for president in 2008 on a platform of change in Washington, D.C. Just as President Obama had spoken for needed change away from the status quo, so did Scott Brown. What resonated with the people of Massachusetts was that change was needed to stop the gridlock in Washington.

What happened with health care reform was basically similar to a football game. The ball had been driven downfield to the one yard line through the coordinated efforts of many people, including the House of Representatives and the United States Senate, and the president of the United States and his administration. But health care reform was stopped by a bone-jarring tackle by newly elected Senator Scott Brown. Some people say, "This is the Scott that was heard around the world." (1) This sent a terrifying chill up the spines of Democrats in both the House and the Senate and sent a very strong message across America in regards to health care reform. Health care reform was now toxic, poisonous, and suicidal to try and continue to push forward. It seemed that the messaging of the Republican Party and their consistent diet of "no" had won, and Democrats were running for the hills.

This speaks to the power of politics to trump the power of policy. Culture beats strategy every time and the culture had changed. What was good for multiple generations of people in finally getting health care headed in a better direction for the nation as a whole now became a symbol of fear of change, government intervention and a massive cost to an already growing deficit. In essence, the Republicans had won. The messaging they had delivered was more convincing and more on target than the Democrats. That has traditionally been the case in Republican politics as their base is a more aligned constituency with similar thinking. The Democrats have always struggled with a much more diverse and broad base, which is harder to message to. The consistent litany messaged by the Republicans of cost, governmental control, harming Medicare, death panels, and fear of the government had simply won out.

The Democrats were in disarray. They could have gone to an immediate conference committee to try to get a final bill passed. However, they opted not to do that, as the power of continuing to upset the American people and the fear of that backlash and what it meant to them in the 2010 midterm elections became an important modifier to their behavior. Senator Harry Reid and Representative Nancy Pelosi both said that they would not do that. Many felt health care reform was now dead. In fact, it was not dead, but it lay on the ground, unconscious and on life support.

Life was brought back into reform over the ensuing weeks after Senator Brown's election. First, President Obama led the charge in his State of the Union address, eight days later, on the 27th of January 2010. In his address to Congress and the American people, President Obama stated that the health care problem in our nation is not going away. He stated that there will be continued loss of people's health insurance and millions will lose it this year. He stated that our deficit will grow, premiums will go up, and patients will be denied the care they need. Small business owners will continue to drop coverage altogether. President Obama stated, "I will not walk away from these Americans, and neither should the people in this chamber." He went on to say, "Here's what I ask Congress, though: don't walk away from reform. Not now. Not when we are so close. Let us find a way to come together and finish the job for the American people. Let's get it done. Let's get it done." (2)

Since the Senate had locked up its 41st vote against healthcare reform, the House of Representatives had one of four options:

1. Let health care reform die.

2. Pass the Senate bill, and go to the president to sign it into law.

3. Pass the Senate bill with House amendments under budget reconciliation. This arcane approach must show cost savings to the federal government, but would then allow further consideration by the Senate of these House amendments. By so doing only a simple majority vote of 51 U.S. Senators would be needed to pass the final bill with the House amendments.

4. Try to pass smaller bills that were more bipartisan in nature.

What then ensued over the next two months was a reemergence of strategies around how to get a healthcare reform bill passed.

President Obama injected himself further into the discussions to try to bridge the gap between the House and the Senate and between Republicans and Democrats. In this effort, President Obama put forth his own health care reform proposal. His proposal was based on three principles. Number one, *affordability*—President Obama wanted to reduce health insurance premiums to tens of millions of families and to help over 32 million Americans afford health care who do not get it today. Under his plan, 95 percent of Americans would be insured. Number two, *accountability*—President Obama wanted to lay down commonsense rules to keep these lower premiums and to prevent insurance industry abuses and denial of care. Specifically, the president wanted to end discrimination against any people with preexisting conditions and to stop denials of care when people need it the most. Number three, *accessibility*—President Obama's plan was to provide a new, competitive, health insurance market, giving tens of millions of Americans the same access and choices to health insurance that members of Congress have.

President Obama also wanted to control costs to help put the nation's budget and our economy on a more stable path. He projected that the health care reform bill should be priced less than 1 trillion dollars and should reduce the deficit by over a hundred billion dollars over the next 10 years and by over a trillion dollars over the second decade (3). Additional targeted policies in the president's proposal were to eliminate the Nebraska Federal Medicaid Assistance Program special provision and to ensure that *all* states receive significant additional funding to expand their Medicaid programs. He also wanted to close the Medicare prescription drug "donut hole" gap and to strengthen the provisions to fight fraud, waste, and abuse in the Medicare and Medicaid programs. President Obama targeted increasing the threshold on the excise tax, for the most expensive health insurance plans from $23,000 for a family plan to $27,500 for a family plan.

President Obama was relentless in his efforts to get the message out to the American people, and made multiple visits from

Pennsylvania to Ohio to Virginia to get this done. He also convened a White House Summit on health care reform, a bipartisan event between important senators and representatives around issues of how to move reform forward. Unfortunately this bipartisan summit did not render any bipartisan support but only confirmed the entrenched nature of both camps. This became a visceral war over the politics of victory or defeat. The Republicans had not forgotten that with the passage of Social Security in 1935 the Democrats rode the popularity of this program for the next 17 years. They desperately did not want to see President Obama and the Democrats get health care reform passed that might ensure 20 years of future success for the Democrats. At all costs, the Republicans wanted a "no vote" on health care reform to successfully provide President Obama his "Waterloo" and bolster their hopes and opportunities for gains in the 2010 midterm elections and the 2012 presidential election. The Democrats, if they failed, would be perceived as not being able to get the job done and would suffer for this in the midterm elections as well. In many ways, it became a no-win situation for the Democrats. If health care reform did not pass, they are seen as being incapable and ineffective in getting the job done. If health care reform passes, they will be branded with all of its failures for the next 20 years unless absolute perfection ensues. Health care reform had been painted as an albatross and hung around the necks of the Democrats for good or for bad. How sad it is for our country to have something as important as the health care of the American people and future generations to be held hostage to the petty principals of politics, fear, change, and the special interests of the status quo.

The United States House of Representatives, which had passed its reform bill on November 7th by a vote of 220 to 215, needed 216 votes to now pass the Senate bill. In the middle of March 2010, much work was done behind the scenes to try to muster these votes. The strategy that the House employed was to use budget reconciliation. Budget reconciliation is a process by which a simple majority vote of 51 votes in the Senate, as opposed to the supermajority vote of 60 votes, can be used when considering bills that have only budgetary implications. On the first day of spring of 2010, the House entered a weekend session to complete action on a companion bill that modified the Senate-passed health care overhaul bill the Patient Protection and Affordable Care Act (H.R.3590). House Democratic leaders worked on this new reconciliation bill known as the Healthcare and Education Affordability Reconciliation Act (H.R.4872). This bill was adamantly opposed by all Republican legislators and by some conservative Democratic representatives. The Congressional Budget Office priced H.R.4872 at $940 billion over the next 10 years. The CBO estimated 138 billion dollars in deficit savings over the first 10 years. This bill then met the criteria required for a budgetary reconciliation bill. Therefore, on March 21, 2010, a Sunday afternoon in Washington, D.C., the biggest health care vote since the 1965 Medicare bill began.

On the evening of March 21, 2010, after more than a year of debate on health care reform, the United States House of Representatives passed H.R.3590, the Patient Protection and Affordable Care Act. The final vote on this bill was 219 to 212. Much wrangling took place for the House to come up with these votes. However, there could have been more votes for this if needed and if it was in serious jeopardy of not passing. The speaker of the house allowed Democrats in very conservative districts to vote their conscience on this bill, in order to keep as much peace as possible with their constituency. Therefore, only enough votes were mustered by the House Democrats to ensure H.R.3590 was passed. The Patient Protection and Affordable Care Act then went to President Obama for signing into law. On March 23, 2010, President Obama signed the Senate bill that had been passed on December 24, 2009, and now passed by the House on March 21, 2010 into law. This bill now became Public Law 111-148 and titled the Patient Protection and Affordable Care Act (PPACA) that I will reference from this point forward by its more common and shortened name of the Affordable Care Act (ACA). During the signing ceremony, President Obama said, "Today, after almost a century of trying; today, after over a year of debate; today, after all the votes have been tallied—health insurance reform becomes law in the United States of America." (4)

On March 21, 2010 the House also passed H.R.4872, known as the Health Care and Education Reconciliation Act of 2010. This was a companion bill to H.R.3590 that contained the amendments, corrections and modifications of H.R.3590 by the United States House of Representatives. This was the bill that used the budget reconciliation process. The intent of the companion bill H.R.4872 was to make changes in Senate bill H.R.3590 that, according to House Democrats, helped strengthen the bill. This bill passed later in the evening by a vote of 220 to 211. It should be noted that neither of the bills passed on the evening of Sunday, March 21, 2010 received any Republican votes. Not one vote. Thirty-three Democrats joined Republicans in opposing the reconciliation bill H.R.4872. Thirty-four Democrats joined with Republicans in voting against Senate bill H.R.3590.

While H.R.3590 went to President Obama for signature, the Senate on March 23, 2010 started to debate H.R.4872. On March 25, 2010, the Senate passed the amended reconciliation bill by a vote of 56 to 43. All Democratic Senators except three voted to pass the amended reconciliation bill. Every Republican again voted against H.R.4872. The bill was then sent back to the House because of two unrelated minor amendments made by the Senate in unrelated educational provisions. The vote in the House on March 26, 2010 was 220 to 207 to pass the Senate amended H.R.4872 Healthcare and Education Act of 2010 on to President Obama for his signature. President Obama signed this companion bill with House amendments, H.R.4872, into law on March 30, 2010.

The signing of these two bills into law by President Obama thus ended one of the most contentious debates in the history of our country. Although this bill is certainly not perfect in every provision, it marks a starting point for continued reform in our health care system that is long overdue. Both the Democrats and the Republicans agree that our health care system is in dire need of reform. What became the contentious points around health care reform legislation however, had more to do with politics than it did around health care policy.

Let's now look in some detail at the final Patient Protection and Affordable Care Act (or as I will refer to it the Affordable Care Act or ACA), by dividing this complex law into its six major pillars, just as we did in Chapter 8 when we reviewed the originally proposed House and Senate bills. As a reminder, these six pillars were:

1. Expansion of coverage

2. Delivery/workforce reform

3. Cost control and financing

4. Health insurance reform

5. Quality reforms

6. Focus on prevention and wellness

A very thorough review of the Affordable Care Act can be found on the Kaiser Family Foundation website (5).

FIRST PILLAR: EXPANSION OF COVERAGE

Percent of Americans Covered/Number Uninsured

The ACA will increase the percentage of U.S. citizens and legal residents covered by health insurance to approximately 94 percent. This will add about 32 million people to insurance programs, decreasing the number of uninsured Americans by about 23 million by the year 2019.

Individual Mandate

The individual mandate is one of the most controversial provisions in the new ACA, requiring that all U.S. citizens and legal residents have health coverage. In fact, at least 26 states are suing the United States government over the constitutionality of requiring an individual mandate. Under the new ACA, the individual mandate will be phased in between the years 2014 and 2016. Under this law individuals must buy insurance or pay a penalty that would be the greater of $695 per year ($2,850 per family), or 2.5 percent of household income. These penalties will be smaller in 2014 and 2015 and the maximum amount will occur in 2016. After 2016, the penalty amount will increase annually by a cost of living adjustment. There will be exemptions granted for financial hardship, religious objections, Native Americans, those without coverage for less than three months, undocumented immigrants, incarcerated individuals, and those with incomes below the tax filing threshold of $9,354 for singles and $18,700 for couples.

Employer Mandate

The Senate bill did not include an employer mandate but did require companies with 50 or more employees to help defray the cost of taxpayers footing the bill for their workers' insurance. This was modified, however, by the reconciliation bill, so that ACA now assesses employers that do not offer coverage and employ more than 50 people a fee of $2,000 annually per full-time employee, excluding the first 30 employees from the assessment. This law becomes effective January 1, 2014. Employers with less than 50 employees would be exempt. There is also a provision that requires employers to provide a free-choice voucher to employees with incomes less than 400 percent of the federal poverty level (FPL), and whose share of the premiums exceed 8 percent but does not exceed 9.8 percent of their income, or who choose to enroll in another plan in the exchange period. The voucher would be equal to what the employer would have paid for coverage under the employer's plan. The intent is to maximize the employee's freedom of choice of health insurance. Employers with more than 200 employees will be required to automatically enroll all employees into the employer-offered health care plan. Employees, however, may still opt out of coverage for another plan in the exchange.

Medicaid Expansion

The new ACA will expand Medicaid to all individuals under the age of 65 with incomes at or below 133 percent of the federal poverty level (FPL). This will start on January 1, 2014 and will include children, pregnant women, parents, and adults without dependent children. Undocumented immigrants are not eligible. The reconciliation bill modified existing law to help states address their concerns about the cost of expanding Medicaid by increasing the federal share of covering newly eligible people. It provides states with 100 percent federal funding for 2014 through 2016. Another major provision added under the reconciliation bill will be that all primary care doctors (family physicians, general internal medicine physicians, or general pediatricians) will have Medicaid rates increased to 100 percent of the Medicare payment rates for 2013 and 2014 in order to help patients have increased access to primary care physicians and avoid the problem seen earlier in Massachusetts. States will receive 100 percent federal financing for this increased payment rate. The reconciliation bill also jettisoned the special deal that several states such as Nebraska, Florida, and Louisiana had secured.

States must also maintain current income eligibility levels for the State Children's Health Insurance Program (SCHIP) until 2019 and extend their funding for SCHIP through 2015. There is already federal assistance for the SCHIP program, but there will be additional federal funding support beginning in 2015.

Health Insurance Exchanges

The ACA creates state-based American health benefit exchanges and Small Business Help Options Program (SHOP) exchanges, administered by either a non-profit organization or a governmental agency.

This will allow individuals and small businesses with up to 100 employees to search, find, and purchase qualified coverage. The new law will allow businesses with more than 100 employees to use the SHOP exchange beginning in 2017. States will be allowed to have more than one exchange in their state based on geography. Funding for states to set up these exchanges will begin within one year of law passage up until January 1, 2015. These exchanges will only serve U.S. citizens and legal immigrants.

Individual Subsidies

The ACA creates premium and cost-sharing subsidies to individuals. The premium credits will be for U.S. citizens and legal immigrants with incomes between 133 percent and 400 percent of the federal poverty level to help them purchase insurance through the exchanges. This will be tied to a sliding fee scale based on percentages of income based on the FPL. Similarly, the cost-sharing subsidies will be provided to eligible individuals and families based on their income level as compared to the federal poverty level. There will need to be verification of both income and citizenship status in determining eligibility for these subsidies. These provisions are aimed at helping individuals and families with lower incomes to be able to afford health insurance coverage.

Public Plan Option

There is no public plan option in the ACA. The senate bill never contained this provision. The original House bill did. The House leadership decided not to try and put a public plan option in the reconciliation bill as they believed there would not be the votes to support this on the Democrats side. The new ACA contains language from the Senate bill that requires the Office of Personnel Management to contract with insurers to offer at least two multistate plans in each exchange. At least one of the plans must be offered by a non-profit entity and at least one plan must not provide coverage for abortions except in the case of rape, incest, or life-threatening condition to the mother. Each of the multistate plans must be licensed in each state.

The creation of these multistate plans is to increase competition in states, based on cost and quality for health insurance plans. Many states and regions have very limited carrier choice, which creates unfair pricing to employers, employees, and individuals. It also sets up unfair dynamics in negotiating contracts with providers. This enhanced competition across state lines is seen as a mitigating factor in place of a federally run public plan option that would have provided competition to these health insurance companies. The result is that private health insurance companies will have increased competition against one another.

Consumer Operated and Oriented Plan (CO-OP)

The ACA establishes consumer operated and oriented plans (CO-OP) through the creation of non-profit, member-run health insurance companies in all 50 states and the District of Columbia to increase competition, choice, and variety for employers, employees, and individuals. These co-ops must have a strong consumer focus and must use any profits made to lower premiums, improve benefits, or improve the quality of healthcare delivered to its members. Six billion dollars will be used to finance the program and award loans and grants to establish CO-OPs by July 1, 2013.

Abortion Coverage

The new law ensures that federal premiums or cost-sharing subsidies are not used to purchase coverage for abortion unless it is for rape, incest, or saving the life of the mother (the long-standing Hyde Amendment). Firewalls were created to ensure that an individual who received individual federal subsidies and purchased a plan in which other abortion services were provided could not use federal subsidy funds to purchase the abortion. President Obama signed an Executive Order on March 24, 2010 making those provisions clear. He did so in an attempt to ensure that critical House Democrats would vote to pass the Senate bill so the nation could move forward on health care reform.

Benefit Package

The ACA creates comprehensive basic health benefits that all qualified health insurance plans must meet. This is where the basic provisions of comprehensive primary care, wellness, prevention, immunizations, and health-focused activities will reside. The secretary of HHS will define and annually update the benefits package through a transparent and public process. This will become effective on January 1, 2014. There will also be a provision for states to create a basic health plan for uninsured individuals that contain this basic benefits package and who make between 133 percent and 200 percent of the federal poverty level. If individuals in a state choose the state's basic health plan, they will not be eligible for subsidies in the exchange. States will be permitted to prohibit plans in the exchange from providing coverage for abortions (except those for rape, incest, or life-threatening maternal condition) if that state so desires.

Benefit Categories

The ACA creates four benefit categories of plans as well as a distinct and separate catastrophic plan. These four basic plans are the bronze, silver, gold, and platinum plans. These four plans offer the essential health benefits package described above and vary only in the percent of the benefit costs of the plan. They limit out-of-pocket spending to that equal with Health Savings Account (HSA) current law, which is $5,950 for individuals and $11,900 for families. The bronze plan covers 60 percent, the silver plan covers 70 percent, the gold plan 80 percent, and the platinum plan covers 90 percent. The catastrophic plan is a separate plan available to those up to the age of 30 or those who are exempt from the mandate to purchase coverage. It provides catastrophic coverage only, but also will make prevention benefits and coverage for three primary care visits exempt from the deductible. The catastrophic plan will only be available in the individual market.

So in summary, the expanded coverage portion of the ACA

provides 32 million more Americans insurance coverage. This will be done through individual and employer mandates and by an expansion of the Medicaid program. Coverage for half of the 32 million newly included will come from Medicaid expansion. Federal subsidies will be used for individuals up to 400 percent of the federal poverty level on a sliding fee scale to help them purchase health care insurance. The expansion of coverage will start primarily in 2014. Including this expansion in coverage, the ACA in total applies to approximately 94 percent of all American citizens.

Now let's turn our attention to the next large pillar of health care reform that became law.

SECOND PILLAR: DELIVERY/WORKFORCE REFORM

It is sad that at a time that we have expanded coverage to 32 million more Americans, that we really do not have the correct physician infrastructure in place to easily meet this demand. Therefore, much attention must be paid to getting the delivery and workforce side of this equation fixed. This is one of the most inadequately addressed areas in all of the new health care reform law. However, there are some very important provisions in the new law to start America down the right track.

Advisory Committee on Health Workforce

The ACA establishes a multi-stakeholder Workforce Advisory Committee, empowered to develop a national workforce strategy. The law called for appointments to be made to this committee by September 30, 2010. Our country has never regulated the types of physicians that America produces. Instead, we leave this important decision in the hands of young medical students. The American Association of Medical Colleges (AAMC) has walked away from their responsibility and accountability to help America with this important issue of creating a physician workforce that meets the nation's needs. Because of this, we have a totally unregulated workforce where many physicians are making their career choices of what type of physician to become more around money and lifestyle than on service and community need. Unfortunately, this funding was held up in Congress. So even after all the committee members were selected, they have never met as a group because the money was not appropriated by Congress. It is unbelievable that a measure as low cost and important as setting a coordinated and long overdue set of policies and principles around workforce is prevented from occurring by continued shortsightedness and preservation of the status quo.

Primary Care and General Surgeon Payment

The ACA will not only increase Medicaid payment to equal that of Medicare payment for primary care doctors for 2013 and 2014 but it also provides a 10 percent payment increase to primary care physicians bills in Medicare for five years beginning January 1, 2011 and running through 2015. This is done to value the services provided by primary care physicians and to start closing the income gap and disparity between primary care physicians and subspecialty physicians and to ensure greater access for patient care. There will also be payment increases for general surgeons who practice in underserved areas, which is also of great community need.

Graduate Medical Education (GME) Redistribution

The new law increases GME residency training positions by redistributing currently unused residency slots, with priorities given to primary care and general surgery residents. States with the lowest resident physician-to-population ratio will have the highest priority. This became effective July 1, 2011. The redistribution will increase the number of residents trained in the primary care areas of family medicine, internal medicine, and general pediatrics as well as in general surgery. This is important in trying to develop a more balanced workforce and to ensure better patient access with what America needs.

Promote Outpatient Training

There must be a reemphasis on training away from monolithic teaching hospitals and out into communities and clinics where patients receive much of their care. The ACA promotes training in outpatient settings by increasing the flexibility and regulations that govern GME funding through Medicare. This became effective July 1, 2010.

Teaching Health Centers

The ACA establishes teaching health centers (THCs), defined as community-based, ambulatory patient care centers, including federally qualified health centers and other federally funded health centers. These THCs are eligible for Medicare payments for the expenses associated with operating primary care residency programs. This began in 2010 with 11 new centers selected in 2011. These centers are much needed models that start to get away from medical and nursing schools as the only places that medical, nursing, and other health-oriented training occurs. These THCs will provide training of teams in community settings where they are the most needed and serve the broader community's needs in an accessible, timely, high-quality, and lower-cost setting.

Scholarship and Loan Repayment

The new law establishes scholarships and loans to support the necessary primary care training and workforce capacity building demanded by the current pressing need to increase the number of primary care physicians. Scholarships will be aimed primarily at increasing recruitment on the front end of medical school into primary care areas. Loan repayments will kick in after residency training to help promote the launch of the new primary care physicians. This is intended to help distribute these physicians to much needed areas in the United States by paying off medical school loans accrued by them. State grants will also be available to providers in medically underserved areas and rural areas. The new law also establishes a public health workforce loan repayment program and will provide medical residents with training in preventive medicine and public health.

Support Primary Care Training

The ACA supports the development of training programs that focus on primary care. In particular, training that supports the new models of the patient-centered medical home, team management of chronic disease, and models that integrate physical and mental health services will be highly encouraged and supported. This funding will be for five years starting in the year 2010.

Mental, Behavioral, and Oral Health Training

The new law supports the development of interdisciplinary mental and behavioral health training programs. There will be further development of training programs for oral health professionals. Again, the purpose is to create much needed increases in underdeveloped parts of our health care workforce. These efforts will not only increase these important workforce elements, but they will also integrate them more tightly together so that more of these services are coordinated.

Expand Nurse Training

Nurses are critical to our future health care system. The anticipated nursing shortage is 2 million nurses over the next 20 years. The ACA increases the capacity for education, training, and retention of nurses. There will also be loan repayment and retention grants. This will be very important to building the health care team we must have to care for both a growing and aging America.

Nurse-Managed Health Clinics

The law created grants for up to three years to federally qualified health centers and nurse managed health clinics to employ and provide training to family nurse practitioners whom will provide primary care in those settings. This is being done in an effort to immediately amplify the front-end funnel of primary care so there are enough providers to handle the increased number of people who will be covered with health care insurance. These funds were provided in 2011 and will run for five years.

Patient-Centered Medical Homes/Integrated Teams

The ACA promotes training in and the provision of integrated and coordinated care through the patient-centered medical home. This is both a place and process of care where leveraging the trusted patient-physician relationship with a team-based approach provides high-quality preventive, acute, and chronic care. It is exactly this model that will start to control cost, improve access, and increase quality of care. Robust primary care has been shown to do this in all other industrialized countries of the world.

Community Health Centers (CHCs)/School-Based Health Centers

The ACA calls for $12 billion for community health centers over a five-year time period starting in 2011. The intent of this is to immediately create, expand, and improve primary care access so that patients have the right places to go for care and the right types of health care providers to see when they get there. The same part of the law supports school-based health centers and nurse managed health clinics, and began in 2010 to help with the immediate access issues to primary care. These funds to date have sadly been curtailed by Congress with only $14 million of this $12 billion being funded.

Public Health and Disaster Preparedness

The ACA commissions a regular corps and the Ready Reserve Corps of trained medical providers for service in times of a national emergency. This helps better prepare our nation proactively for these emergencies and gets us away from a reactive, chaotic response as we have seen in the past (e.g., Hurricane Katrina and the devastation of New Orleans).

Trauma Care

The reconciliation bill added trauma care to the new ACA. The law establishes new trauma center programs to strengthen emergency department and trauma center capacity. This law will also fund research and innovative models for emergency care systems. This will help provide better, more-efficient, and effective catastrophic care. These funds started in 2011.

American Indians

The ACA immediately reauthorized and amended the Indian Health Care Improvement Act. This became effective immediately upon bill passage. This allows America's original citizens to have ongoing universal health care with no bills, similar to that provided by the Veterans Affairs (VA) and the Department of Defense (DOD) military health system.

So in summary, the ACA was designed to immediately start working on building the necessary workforce our nation needs for our future. It was designed to do so by standing up a National Workforce Commission that would advise Congress, the president, HHS, HRSA, and others on a workforce strategy that will form a firm foundation for the types of physicians and other health care professionals our nation will need. This unhappily was mothballed by the 112th Congress and thus frozen by not appropriating funding. The ACA is designed to rebuild the important primary care and general surgery workforce by valuing their important contributions and by paying them more for their much-needed services. It also incentivizes those going into primary care through scholarships and loan repayment programs. The workforce/delivery provisions also call for different models of care and locations of care that support accessible, integrated primary care provided by coordinated teams of providers.

THIRD PILLAR: COST CONTROL AND FINANCING

One of the most contentious issues in health care reform was cost. At a time with rapidly growing national debt and a burgeoning national deficit, many asked how can we continue to spend more? The Congressional Budget Office (CBO) estimates that the ACA will cost $938 billion over 10 years. The costs are to be paid for through a combination of savings from Medicare and Medicaid, as well as new taxes and fees. What is often forgotten, however, is that the Congressional Budget Office estimates that the new law will reduce the deficit by $124 billion over the next 10 years, from what the projected health care costs would have been if left unchanged, and over $1 trillion over the next 10 years after that (6).

Considering that $2.6 trillion is spent each year on health care in the United States, $938 billion over 10 years is an incredibly good investment, one that in fact can actually reduce the deficit long term, while providing our nation higher-quality, greater access, and improved long-term health care. For the cost of only $93.8 billion per year, we significantly begin to reign in our very expensive health care industry. When compared to the $2.6 trillion per year we now spend on health care, this represents only 3.6 percent of our annual health care expenditure.

The key point here is that the new health care reform law starts to control cost as opposed to adding new expense to the growing deficit of our already beleaguered economy. This is an investment in our nation's future economic health as well as physical and mental health.

Medicare Cost Control

Enacting major health care reform and cost savings in Medicare provides the largest incentives because it targets the most expensive utilizers of the health care system, the elderly, and, in particular, the sick elderly. Medicare becomes the lynch pin of health care reform. What happens with Medicare cost control and fee-setting tends to ripple in the private sector as the gold standard. Therefore, gaining control over the cost of Medicare becomes pivotal to controlling and reforming America's health care costs.

- **Medicare Advantage Plans**: The ACA restructures payments to the Medicare Advantage plans (MA). These high-end Medicare insurance plans are traditionally 14 percent higher than the basic Medicare plan. The problem is that private health insurance companies that market these high-end Medicare Advantage plans are paid those extra payments by the federal government and make quite a bit of profit for the administration of these plans. The federal government wants to dial down the cost of what it is paying to private insurance companies to administer these plans and will phase in revised payments over three to six years, which began in 2011. There were also bonus provisions based on quality of care versus just quantity of care.

- **Innovation Center**: The new law creates an Innovation Center within the Centers for Medicare and Medicaid Services to test, evaluate, and expand different models of care that will maximize quality and reduce cost. This will apply to programs in Medicare, Medicaid, and SCHIP and was effective on January 1, 2011. Albert Einstein once said that the definition of insanity is doing the same thing over and over again and expecting a different outcome. We must change the model if we want to affect higher quality and lower cost. This new Innovation Center starts to do this.

- **Reduce Preventable Hospital Readmissions**: In order to maximize coordination and integration of care, patients upon discharge from the hospital need to be reseen by their primary care physician to continue their care and help prevent readmission. In order to make sure that coordinated hand-off and transition occurs, Medicare will reduce payments to hospitals if this does not happen. The exact amount is yet to be determined. Effective date will be October 1, 2012.

- **Reduce Medicare Disproportionate Share Hospital Payments (DSH)**: The new law will reduce hospital payments for what is named Medicare disproportionate share hospital payments. This is an amount of money that has typically been paid to hospitals that see an inordinately large number of uninsured and Medicaid patients to help offset uncompensated care. With more people being covered by health insurance, these payments will be initially cut by 75 percent. Thereafter, there will be increase payments back to these hospitals based on the number of uninsured and the amount of uncompensated care they provide. This will become effective in 2014.

- **Accountable Care Organizations (ACO)**: The new law will allow providers in accountable care organizations (ACOs) to share in cost savings to the Medicare system by better coordinating and integrating care. These organizations must meet certain quality standards and be accountable for the overall care of the Medicare beneficiaries. They must demonstrate adequate participation of primary care physicians, utilize evidence-based medicine, and report on quality, costs, and demonstrated coordination of care. This program went into effect in January 2012.

- **Medicare Part D Subsidies**: The law tightens up Medicare Part D (drug program). Those Medicare Part D beneficiaries with incomes over $85,000 as an individual and $170,000 as a couple will have a reduction in premium subsidies for the Medicare drug program. This will provide subsidy relief to those most in need and exclude those who can afford not to have this subsidy at the federal government's expense. This law became active on January 1, 2011. It is the first step into Medicare means testing to determine how much of the full benefit people should receive based on income.

- **Medicare Part B Premium Freeze**: The new law will freeze the threshold for Medicare Part B premiums for Medicare patients so that new increases in premiums to Medicare recipients will not occur for physician coverage. This became effective January 1, 2011 and extends through 2019.

- **Independent Payment Advisory Board (IPAB)**: The new law creates an Independent Payment Advisory Board, which will consist of 15 members who will submit legislative proposals with recommendations to reduce the per capita growth rate in Medicare spending if spending exceeds target growth rates. This is a mechanism by which Medicare can control its rate of spending and growth by expert opinion and try to depoliticize Medicare cuts. Medicare per capita spending is tied to the gross domestic product per capita and will cause the Board to submit recommendations if this spending exceeds GDP per capita plus 1 percent. These recommendations will go to the president and to Congress. The board will be prohibited from rationing care, increasing revenues, or changing benefits, eligibility, or Medicare beneficiary cost sharing. Hospitals and hospices were given exemptions through the year 2019 and clinical labs for one year. These exemptions keep them from being subjected to cost reductions. These exemptions were not looked upon favorably by the rest of the health care industry. How can hospitals, which are the largest utilizer of Medicare spending, be exempt from cost control for almost a decade? The IPAB will submit recommendations every other year to slow the growth in national health expenditures while preserving quality of care, starting by January 1, 2015.

- **Hospital-Acquired Conditions:** The new law calls for a reduction in Medicare payments to hospitals in which patients in these hospitals develop certain hospital-acquired conditions such as urinary tract infections, blood clots in legs, or pneumonia acquired from being on a ventilator. This reduction will start in the year 2015 and will amount to about 1 percent of that hospital's Medicare payments.

Medicaid Cost Reductions

The Medicaid program that provides care to those with incomes of less than 133 percent of the federal poverty level also has three major provisions for cost reductions.

- **Medicaid Disproportionate Share Hospitalizations (DSH):** The new law will start to reduce the amount of Medicaid disproportionate share hospitalization allotments by $18.1 billion by the year 2020. This will start with a $0.5 billion reduction in 2014 and will be $0.6 billion in the years 2015 and 2016, $1.8 billion in 2017, $5 billion in 2018, $5.6 billion in 2019, and $4 billion in 2020. The methodology will be applied so that the largest reductions in DSH allotments will occur in states with the lowest percentage of uninsured. The rationale for this is that as more and more people have some sort of health care insurance and coverage, there will need to be less apportionment by the federal government to help hospitals with these cost write-offs.

- **Hospital-Acquired Health Care Conditions:** The new law will prohibit federal payments to states for Medicaid services for certain hospital-acquired health care conditions similar to the Medicare program. This will become effective July 1, 2011.

- **Medicaid Drug Rebate Program:** The new law will increase the Medicaid drug rebate percentage for brand-name drugs to 23 percent; percent reduction for other drugs will range from 13 to 17 percent of the average manufacturer price. This law became active upon signature by President Obama.

New Revenue Sources

The new health care reform law brings many tax increases that are related to health insurance for the financing of health reform.

- **Medicare Part A Hospital Insurance**: The new law increases the Medicare Part A (hospital insurance) tax rate on earned income by 0.9 percent. This increase is from 1.45 percent to 2.35 percent on individuals who earn over $200,000 or $250,000 for married couples filing jointly. Additionally, there is a 3.8 percent tax on unearned income for higher income tax payers. This becomes effective on January 1, 2013.

- **Excise Tax on Expensive Insurance Policies**: The new law creates an excise tax on insurers of employer-sponsored health plans that exceed $10,200 for individual coverage or $27,500 for family coverage. These taxes were imposed on high-end insurance policies that tend to promote overutilization of health care by the system. Insurers are the ones penalized and not the persons who purchase the plans. This provision became controversial through the health care reform debates from both the health insurance and unions perspectives. To meet these concerns the date for implementation was pushed back to the year 2020. This in part is what led to the perceptions that back room deals on health care reform were used to get the bill passed.

- **Annual Fees on Pharmaceutical Industry**: The new law increases annual fees paid to the federal government by the pharmaceutical manufacturing industry. This will amount to

$2.8 billion in the years 2012 and 2013; $3 billion in 2014 through 2016; $4 billion in 2017; $4.1 billion in 2018; and $2.8 billion in 2019 and beyond.

- **Annual Fees on Health Insurance Sector**: The health insurance sector also have been assessed annual fees. These will be assessed as follows: $8 billion in 2014; $11.3 billion in 2015 through 2016; $13.9 billion in 2017; $14.3 billion in 2018. Thereafter, the fee amount will be that paid in the previous year increased by the rate of the premium growth.

- **Excise Tax on Medical Devices:** Starting in the year 2013, the new law imposes an excise tax of 2.3 percent on the sale of any taxable medical device.

- **Indoor Tanning Services**: The new law imposes a 10 percent tax for people utilizing indoor tanning services. This was done since these tanning parlors increase people's risk of skin cancers, so these services were levied a health-related tax similar to tobacco companies. This law became effective on July 10, 2010.

Administrative Simplification

Much needs to be done to simplify the complex patchwork of forms and paperwork and computer work of the business of health care. It is a system that is out of control in regards to redundancies, duplications, and inefficiencies. The new law simplifies health insurance administration as noted below:

- **Single Set of Operating Rules**: The creation of a single set of operating rules to determine eligibility verification and claim status were adopted by July 1, 2011. These operating rules will become effective on January 1, 2013.

- **Electronic Funds Transfers**: A system for electronic fund transfers to physicians, hospitals, and other health care providers for health care payment will have rules adopted by July 1, 2012. These electronic fund transfers will become operational on January 1, 2014.

- **Referral Certification and Authorization**: Easy information transmission of referral certification and authorization will occur by means of rules adopted by July 1, 2014, becoming effective on January 1, 2016.

- **Penalties for Noncompliance**: Under the new law, all health plans must document compliance with these standards or face a penalty of no more than $1 per covered life. This will become effective on April 1, 2014.

Eliminate Waste Fraud and Abuse

The ACA calls for enhanced oversight screening and compliance programs to reduce waste, fraud, and abuse. There will also be the creation of a database to share data across federal and state programs, and to increase penalties for submitting false claims. There will be increased funding for anti-fraud activities. These items have various dates in which they become active.

Prescription Drugs

The new law grants new biologic drug manufacturers 12 years of exclusive use before generic versions of biologic drugs can be developed. This was a concession to the pharmaceutical industry to allow them a longer time period (as opposed to the seven years of patent-protected time currently) to make profit on their new drugs. This was in exchange for pharmaceutical industry fees assessed as noted above. The new law authorizes the FDA to approve these generic versions. This law became effective upon the president's signing of the ACA.

In summary, there was much accomplished to begin to bend the cost curve of health care by the Affordable Care Act. These cost reductions amount to approximately $124 billion over the first decade of health care reform and a trillion dollars over the second decade. This will come about through cost reductions in the Medicare and Medicaid programs, administrative simplification, enhanced elimination of waste fraud and abuse, and by new revenue sources. These new sources will be increased taxes on Medicare Part A hospital insurance, on expensive insurance policies, on medical devices, and on indoor tanning services. There will also be annual fees assessed on the pharmaceutical and health insurance sectors to pay for health care reform. When taken together, a good start to meaningful health care reform.

FOURTH PILLAR: HEALTH INSURANCE REFORM

Until we get the health insurance industry operating under guidelines and standards that eliminate discrimination for preexisting conditions, guarantee insurance renewal, have no annual or lifetime caps, stop rescissions for those that become seriously ill, eliminate cost sharing for preventive care, stop gender discrimination, and extend coverage for young adults, we have a wildly out-of-control system. This became one of the most important and defining items in the ACA.

Guaranteed Issue and Rating Rules

All health insurance plans participating in the individual, small group, and exchange markets will be required to provide guaranteed issue and renewability. Allowed rating will only occur based on age, geographic area, family composition, and tobacco use. Required risk adjustment will still occur with all plans that participate. This will begin on January 1, 2014 when the guaranteed issue and rating rules kick in.

Temporary High-Risk Pool

The ACA creates a temporary national high-risk pool to provide health insurance for those U.S. citizens and legal immigrants with preexisting medical conditions who have been uninsured for at least six months. The new law will allow these individuals to be eligible for enrollment in the high-risk pool and to receive subsidized premiums. The law will appropriate $5 billion to finance the program. This became effective 90 days after ACA law enactment and runs until January 1, 2014 when the Guaranteed Issue and Rating Rules kick in. These provisions were put in place to act as a bridge until health insurance exchanges could be developed in each state as a means to ensure that those high-risk patients with complex medical problems would be afforded health insurance coverage.

Medical Loss Ratio and Premium Reviews

The ACA requires health insurance plans to report the proportional amount of premium dollars spent on clinical services, quality, and other costs publicly. If the amount of this spending on clinical services and quality is less than 85 percent of the premium costs (i.e., the medical loss ratio) for the large group market, then these insurers will need to provide rebates to consumers. For plans in the individual and small group markets, these rebates would be paid if this proportional amount is less than 80 percent of the premiums. These two provisions are important as the health insurance industry should be in existence to provide health care payments to the people it covers. If more than 15 cents on every dollar from the large group plans, or 20 cents on every dollar from the individual and small group plans, are being kept by the companies as opposed to plowed back into health care coverage and payment, then these laws will take this extra amount and return it to the customers. This is a very good provision because the medical loss ratio, or the amount paid for clinical services, in Medicare and Medicaid is about 95 to 97 percent, as it is in other industrialized countries. This became effective on January 1, 2011. Also in the ACA will be a process for transparent review of increases in health plan premiums and language around justification of premium increases. There is also a requirement for states to report on premium increase trends. This provision on premium reviews became effective in 2010.

Administrative Simplification

The ACA promotes administrative simplification by the adoption of clear standards for all financial and administrative transactions. This is long overdue. These provisions will help patients, employers, providers, and others finally clearly understand the arcane health insurance system.

Dependent Coverage

The ACA uses the language in the Senate bill, which provides coverage for dependent children up to the age of 26 for all individual and group policies. This became effective six months following the bill becoming law.

Insurance Market Rules

The ACA enacts a standard set of insurance market rules, which prohibit placing lifetime limits on the amount of coverage to people and prohibits insurers from rescissions (i.e., rescinding coverage because one gets a serious illness such as cancer) except in cases of fraud. There was an immediate enactment of prohibiting preexisting condition exclusions for children that became effective six months following enactment of the law. There are also grandfather provisions for existing individual and group plans that require them to extend dependent coverage to age 26, prohibits rescissions of coverage because one gets sick, eliminates waiting periods for coverage to no greater than 90 days, and eliminates lifetime limits and annual limits on coverage. These grandfather plans also eliminated preexisting exclusions for children within six months of enactment and by 2014 for adults. Also in the ACA was a requirement that all new policies comply with one of the four benefit plan categories (i.e., bronze, silver, gold, platinum). There is also a limit on deductibles to $2,000 for individuals and

$4,000 for families, which becomes effective on January 1, 2014 as well. The ACA calls for the creation of the Temporary Reinsurance Program that covers high-risk individuals (i.e., "high-risk pools"). This high-risk re-insurance program will be financed by mandatory contributions from the health insurers totaling $25 billion over three years, which becomes effective January 1, 2014 through December 2016. Finally, the ACA allows states the options of merging individual and small group markets as they see fit.

Consumer Protections

The new law established Internet websites to identify health care coverage options using standard formats, effective on July 1, 2010. It also developed standards for insurers to provide information on benefits and coverage that are clear and understandable within 12 months following enactment.

Selling Insurance Across State Lines

The ACA will permit states to develop health care choice compacts and allow health insurance companies to sell policies in any state that participates in the compact. This will allow for more choice and more options for individuals, small groups, and large groups. There will be a requirement that the coverage must be at least as comprehensive and affordable as coverage provided through the state exchanges. These regulations will be out in 2013, and the compacts will start on or about January 1, 2016.

Health Insurance Administration

The ACA creates the Health Insurance Reform Implementation Fund to be located in the Department of Health and Human Services. The ACA allocates $1 billion to this fund to help the Department of Health and Human Services in the implementation of all of these health reform policies that have been mentioned above.

Requirements of Participating Health Plans

The ACA will require all participating health plans to meet several requirements. They must have adequate provider networks. They must contract with navigators (people who help guide patients through the system) to conduct outreach and enrollment assistance. They must meet accreditation standards for quality measures. They must report in plain language information on claims payment policies, enrollment, disenrollment, number of claims denied, cost-sharing requirements, out-of-network policies, and enrollee rights.

Requirements of Exchanges

The ACA will also ensure that exchanges provide call centers for customer service, provide single application forms, submit financial reports to the secretary of HHS, and provide oversight investigations of the operation and administration of the exchanges.

In summary, these reform measures of the health insurance industry are very important in tightening up a very expensive, inefficient, costly, and under-regulated industry. Many of these provisions start quickly. The creation of the temporary high-risk pool went into effect within six months to allow individuals the ability to purchase health care insurance until the health care insurance exchanges are on line in 2014. By applying equitable consistent standards to stop discriminatory practices regarding rescissions of insurance, annual and lifetime caps, denials of care based on preexisting conditions, and other health insurance practices as noted above, we will finally be able to give to every American a sense of security and stability around their health care programs. Sadly, one item that was not included in the reconciliation bill was the anti-trust exemptions. These exemptions were specifically to remove health insurance and medical malpractice insurers from price setting on health insurance and medical liability prices at both doctors' and patients' expense. This will have to await further legislation down the road.

FIFTH PILLAR: QUALITY REFORMS

As we have talked about earlier in this chapter, we must overhaul coverage, delivery, cost, and our health insurance system. An additional, absolutely critical part of getting a better performing and higher-value health care system is to improve the quality of our health care system. Remember our definition of value. Value equals quality divided by cost. Anything that increases quality in that scenario while holding cost steady will increase value. If quality goes up while cost goes down this really enhances value. The following provisions in the ACA help move us upward on the quality continuum.

National Quality Strategy

The ACA created the National Quality Improvement Strategy. This strategy would include priorities on improvements in health care services delivery, health care outcomes, population health, and the creation and usage of quality measures. This strategy has already been delivered to Congress.

Quality Measures

The ACA created processes and priorities for performance improvement and quality measures that will be developed by multiple stakeholders and will be used in reporting and payment. The Medicare Physician Quality Reporting Initiative (PQRI) is an example of one such program. These quality measures will be utilized for hospitals, clinics, skilled nursing facilities, home health agencies, and ambulatory surgical centers in varying degrees.

Medical Homes

The creation of "medical homes" or "health homes" is a provision in the ACA to integrate and coordinate care through primary care physicians and their practices to improve quality and lower cost. This provision is in the Medicaid state plans and will permit Medicaid patients with at least two chronic conditions, or one condition and risk of developing another, or at least one serious and persistent mental health condition to designate a provider (or a practice) as a "health home." This provision also exists in the law for Medicare patients under the section on innovative models. The medical home/health home model must be applied to all patients in such practices so that the demonstrated quality improvements and cost reductions of primary care, seen in other countries, can be extended to the entire population and not just the chronically ill.

Bundled Payments

The ACA establishes a national Medicare pilot program to develop and evaluate the approach of making bundled payments for acute inpatient hospital services, physician services, outpatient hospital services, and post-acute care services for an episode of care that begin three days prior to a hospitalization and extend to 30 days following discharge. If these programs show improvement in quality and reduction in cost, then these pilot programs will be expanded. These programs will be developed by January 1, 2013. The successful pilots will be extended to January 1, 2016. Under the Medicaid provisions of the ACA, these same episodes of care will be evaluated through such bundled payments or global capitated payments to "safety net" hospital systems. This will also look at the provision of services for pediatric patients and the treatment of mental diseases for adults.

Community-Based Collaborative Care Network

The ACA called for the establishment of this network to help support health care providers in coordinating and integrating health care services. This program is targeted primarily at low income, uninsured, and underinsured populations. The idea here is similar to the old farm agent program that was utilized in every community to help improve the practices of farmers through best practices sharing and education. Similarly, this model could be used for these safety net groups in regards to helping promote higher-quality and lower-cost care. This was to have been a five-year program starting in 2011. Unfortunately, these funds were also not appropriated by the 112th Congress.

Independence at Home Demonstration Program

The ACA created the Independence at Home Demonstration Program to provide high need Medicare beneficiaries primary care services in their home. By integrating and coordinating this care with multiple other members of the team of health professionals that provide this global, comprehensive care, cost savings and quality should occur. This demonstration program would allow the entire team to share in the savings as they show reduction in preventable emergency room visits, hospitalizations, and preventable readmissions to the hospital, while they in parallel improve health care outcomes, improve the efficiency of care, reduce the cost of health care, and improve patient satisfaction. This demonstration program became effective on January 1, 2012.

Hospital-Based Purchasing

The ACA establishes a hospital-based purchasing program in Medicare to pay hospitals based on their ability to deliver certain quality measures. This is aimed at having hospitals strive for a higher quality of care and to be able to both measure and obtain them. It will tie payments to the achievement of these outcomes. This became effective in fiscal year 2012.

Health Care Disparities

One of the major determinants of our poor quality outcomes when measured by international standards is the disparity of care that occurs in our population. This provision of the ACA helps to better understand and to eliminate these disparities. It will require enhanced reporting and collection of data on race, ethnicity, sex, primary language, disability status, and information on underserved rural and frontier populations. This information will be analyzed by the secretary of Health and Human Services, who will examine the data and report on trends and disparities. This will become effective two years following enactment. This measure speaks to the old quality adage of what gets measured gets improved.

Comparative Effectiveness Research

The ACA creates a non-profit Patient-Centered Outcomes Research Institute to help identify research priorities and conduct research that compares the clinical effectiveness of medical treatments. This non-profit institute will be overseen by a Board of Governors be assisted by expert advisory panels. The purpose of this research is to provide evidence-based data to physicians and other health care providers at the point of service and to patients to help in the shared decision making of what treatments, diagnostic testing, and medical approaches are the most appropriate. This will improve quality and lower cost, and thus increase value.

Financial Disclosure

The ACA includes language to ensure that there is required disclosure of financial relationships between health entities to decrease potential conflicts of interest and to ensure that there is no blatant financial gain from the provision of health care. Those being required to disclose will include physicians, hospitals, pharmacists, other providers, manufacturers and distributers of covered drugs, devices, biologicals, and medical supplies. The provision calls for a report to Congress by April 1, 2013.

In summary, the Affordable Care Act helps us advance relatively rapidly down the road of developing a higher-quality and higher-value health care system. It does so by erecting a national quality strategy that prioritizes those measures designed to enhance delivery of health care services, improve health care outcomes, effectively use quality measures, and by doing so improve the population health of the community as a whole. This part of the Affordable Care Act will start to innovate around patient-centered medical homes (PCMHs), accountable care organizations (ACOs), different payment models, community and home care, and decreasing health care disparities. One key area of involvement here will be the applying of comparative effectiveness research to help determine the most effective and efficient way to provide high-quality care at reasonable cost.

SIXTH PILLAR: FOCUS ON PREVENTION AND WELLNESS

As has been mentioned many times throughout this book, our health care system focuses on reactive "sick care" versus proactive health care. It is for this reason that another important part of the ACA focuses on prevention and wellness. There must be incentives and strategies that will move our health care system toward the upstream front end of medicine, wellness, and prevention. It has been seen over the last 40 years that our health care system will not do this by itself. Therefore, proactive steps that mandate and incentivize these sorts of programs and initiatives are paramount.

National Strategy

The ACA established the National Prevention Health Promotion and Public Health Council. The purpose of this council is to coordinate federal prevention, wellness, and public health activities. This council focuses on creating a healthier America. One of the goals of the council is to create a Prevention and Public Health Fund to expand and sustain funding for prevention and public health programs. One of the mechanisms by which this was done was by the creation of task forces on community preventive services.

- **Prevention and Public Health Fund**: This fund was to receive $7 billion in funding for fiscal years 2010 through 2015 and $2 billion for each fiscal year after 2015 to help coordinate activities related to prevention, wellness, public health, and health screenings.

- **Grants Programs**: These grants programs were to focus on the delivery of prevention and wellness services and efforts to reduce chronic disease rates and health disparities. They were to be focused in particular on rural and frontier areas.

Unfortunately, both of these programs and this provision were cannibalized by the 112th Congress as a source of funding for other programs. This shortsighted vision around the importance of prevention is yet again displayed by our Congress.

Prevention Services Coverage

The ACA will help improve prevention by eliminating the burden of cost sharing for preventive services in the Medicare and Medicaid programs. Only those services that have been proven by the United States Preventive Services Task Force (USPSTF) will be covered along with recommended immunizations. Medicare payments for these services will be 100 percent of actual charges for fee schedule rates. This became effective January 1, 2011.

- **Comprehensive Health Risk Assessment**: A comprehensive health risk assessment will be provided to all Medicare beneficiaries upon entry into the Medicare program. This assessment will also include a personalized prevention plan.

- **Behavior Modification Program**: A behavior modification program will be created to provide incentives to both Medicare and Medicaid beneficiaries to help engage these patients in behavioral change. As has been mentioned earlier in the book, 40 percent of all deaths are due to behavioral problems such as obesity, sedentary lifestyles, lack of exercise, smoking, excessive alcohol use, and lack of seat belt utilization, among others. Therefore, incentivizing behavioral change becomes critical to improving health and lowering costs. This program became effective in 2011.

- **Smoking Cessation**: The new law creates tobacco cessation services for pregnant women in the Medicaid program. This became effective in October 2010.

- **Health Plans Coverage**: The ACA requires all qualified health plans to provide minimum coverage without cost sharing for preventive services that have been proven effective by the USPSTF. This also includes recommended immunizations, preventive care for infants, children, and adolescents, and additional preventive care and screenings for women. This became effective six months after signing into law.

Wellness Programs

The ACA was to provide grants for up to five years to small employers to establish wellness programs. This was to begin in fiscal year 2011. This was really important because getting people involved and motivated about wellness will save cost while promoting a healthier workforce and healthier people. The law also provided technical assistance to the employer to provide expertise in setting up and sustaining wellness programs. It also permitted employers to offer rewards of premium discounts up to 30 percent of coverage for employees that participate in these programs and meet certain health standards. The funding for these programs was frozen by the 112th Congress.

Nutrition Information

The ACA requires chain restaurants and food sold from vending machines to disclose nutritional information for each item to educate the public in order to help them make better choices. We are what we eat, and this effort will help promote better health, less obesity, and less long-term downstream chronic diseases.

Preventive Medicine and Public Health Education

The ACA requires graduate medical education residency programs to provide curriculum around preventive care and public health. This is currently being done in the primary care residency disciplines of family medicine, internal medicine, and pediatrics. This requirement, however, will ensure that all physicians in training in all other types of residency programs will have these principles sewn into their education. This will help create better-trained physicians that will start to value the principles of prevention and public health to a larger degree than they do now.

In summary, the Affordable Care Act jumpstarts reform by developing a national strategy for our country in regards to prevention, wellness, and public health. By having a plan in place we will start to integrate and coordinate prevention, wellness, and public health into our new health care system's DNA. We will truly focus on changing behaviors to produce a healthier people and a healthier nation. We as a nation must commit our resources and finances to these important areas of health care reform.

OTHER AREAS OF REFORM

There are other areas contained in the ACA that do not easily fall into these six major pillars. These areas are discussed below.

Medical Malpractice

This is the most striking area of all of the health care reform law that was blatantly omitted. We had a significant opportunity to make major changes in an antiquated and terribly out-of-balance and unregulated medical malpractice environment. This omission caused major consternation among the physician community and between the two political parties. However, the ACA does contain five-year demonstration grants to states to develop, implement, and evaluate alternatives to current tort litigations. These will be aimed at programs that will enhance patient safety and reduce medical errors and adverse events. These innovative programs will look at plans that will improve access to reasonable and affordable liability insurance. Funding for these grants started in fiscal year 2011.

Long-Term Care

The ACA provides a great opportunity to start to proactively look into the provisions of long-term care. America is aging. We have 80 million plus Medicare beneficiaries hitting the books within the next 15 years. The ACA contains several provisions to improve quality while controlling cost in this important area.

The CLASS Act

The ACA establishes the Community Living Assistance Services and Supports Program (CLASS Program). This is a national voluntary insurance program for purchasing coverage. After being vested for five years the program offers a cash benefit of no less than $50 a day to help purchase necessary nonmedical services and support so that individuals can live in their own homes. The program will be funded through voluntary payroll deductions. All working adults will be automatically enrolled unless they opt out. The program was to have become effective January 1, 2011. This program was stopped by the administration because it was determined to be fiscally unsustainable.

Home Care Options

Being able to continue to provide people home care will be important to both their satisfaction as well as cost control. The ACA provides states with new options for offering home and community-based services through Medicaid state plans. This will provide community-based attendant supports and services and create incentive programs to increase the proportion of non-institutionally based long-term care. Another key provision in the ACA is that Medicaid money will follow the person and their needs, and not necessarily go to institutions. These programs run variably from October 1, 2010 to September 30, 2015 for funding.

Skilled Nursing Facility Requirements

In an effort to increase transparency and quality of skilled nursing facilities, the ACA requires these facilities to disclose information regarding ownership, accountability, requirements, and expenditures. All of this information will be placed on a website so that Medicare patients can compare the facilities and make informed choices about a skilled nursing facility (nursing home) for care.

Prescription Medication Coverage

The ACA provides reform around prescription medication coverage for the elderly. There are several provisions that help the elderly with Medicare Part D drug coverage.

- **Medicare Part D Gap Reduction**: The ACA will phase down the beneficiary coinsurance rate in the Medicare Part D coverage gap from 100 percent to 25 percent by the year 2020. This effort will begin to close the so-called donut hole. In addition to this there was a $250 rebate to all Medicare beneficiaries who reach the Part D coverage gap in the year 2010.

- **Brand-Name Medication Cost Reduction**: There was a 50 percent discount on prescriptions filled in the Medicare Part D coverage for brand name drugs. This offset of 50 percent was required by pharmaceutical manufacturers beginning in 2011.

SUMMARY

So there you have it. The Patient Protection and Affordable Care Act (PPACA), more often referred to as the Affordable Care Act (ACA), became the law of our land on March 23, 2010. It is a monumental piece of health care legislation designed to overhaul many aspects of the United States health care system. It targets six major areas of health care in our country: expansion of coverage, delivery/ workforce reform, cost control, health insurance reform, quality reform, and a focus on wellness and prevention. It also includes legislation regarding long-term care, Medicare prescription Part D reform, and early baby steps into medical liability reform.

It may appear to many that the ACA is full of pilot programs. It is, but this is by design. To sow the seeds of innovation and to encourage pioneering solutions requires exploratory programs. This approach is not new to American thinking. We did this with agriculture and farming in the 1900s. Because of pilot programs, ones based on scientific evidence and the sharing of best practices, we transformed farming in our country. One hundred years later, we stand on a similar threshold with health care reform. These pilots will stimulate new thinking that, along with a wise alignment of financial incentives, will revolutionize our American health care system.

What is next in the journey? Consider that in making important decisions, groups will go through a four-part process. The group will form, it will storm, it will norm, and then the group will perform. This is true for nations as well. When a nation takes on an issue as large as health care, it is a mighty undertaking. When a nation confronts a task like health care reform—affecting the largest economic sector in the American economy—everyone takes notice. When a nation tackles a topic that will affect the well-being of every man, woman, and child in this country for the next 100 years, the issue commands deep feelings, beliefs, and values. It also unleashes fear, anger, and deep discomfort.

This amount of angst and turmoil quite honestly is to be expected as our nation "storms" around health care reform, and is a necessary step before our country can move on to the next stages of "norming" and "performing." Clearly for health care reform, the storming is not yet over; and because of the long implementation phase of the ACA over the next decade, the process will be prolonged. There are many who are still deeply bothered by a host of concerns that are as unique as the different parts of the law itself. Most of the passionate dislike centers on the cost of implementing the law; on the perceived shift in control of health care away from states and the private sector into the hands of the federal government; and on the compelling of individuals, the states, or the private sector, to do things they don't want to do. Some examples of this latter concern include the individual mandate to have insurance and the requirement of states to expand Medicaid to more of the poor.

Since the passage of the Affordable Care Act, we have seen considerable storming over its provisions in Congress, particularly in the Republican-dominated House of Representatives that resulted from the power shift caused by the 2010 midterm election. The midterm seat change in the House has led to many efforts to defund, destabilize, or stop many of the provisions of the Affordable Care Act, though the U.S. Senate has strongly indicated it will not support such efforts to repeal or alter the ACA. It is also important to realize that President Obama would likely veto any efforts to dismantle the major provisions of the Affordable Care Act. Meanwhile the constitutional challenge of the Individual Mandate provision in Florida, Virginia, and elsewhere based on the grounds that citizens cannot be forced to purchase health care insurance if they don't want to, has left many people, many states, and our nation wondering what comes next as these cases will soon be acted upon by the Supreme Court.

Our country has now entered an awkward stalemate around health care reform. However, our nation, just like in group dynamics, will eventually move on to "norming" and will eventually come together around the provisions of health care reform. We have already begun this in some ways since the bill's passage. With struggle, our nation will progress to the "performing" stage. The question is: how long will this all take? The unfolding of the storming stage is critically important in answering this. Undoubtedly, the conflict that comes from storming will be necessary before we can as a nation move forward. It should be pointed out that without question, the fate of the 2012 presidential and congressional elections will be critical in defining the direction and speed of future health care reform in our country. But in any case, America will find ways to make health care reform work. Even if the Supreme Court finds the individual mandate unconstitutional much of the Affordable Care Act will be continued because it is such a broad and comprehensive law and most of it is not based on this mandate.

It is similar to being dealt a hand of cards. You may or may not like the hand of cards you have, but that is the hand you have been dealt. It is now incumbent on our nation, our states, and every American to play this hand of cards to the best of our abilities. This is what performing means. We must now make some very important decisions as to whether we are going to make our newly created health care reform law work or not. I can tell you one thing for certain, sooner or later we must reform our health care system or a financial catastrophe with exponentially growing costs will bankrupt us as a nation and rob us of the ability to stay competitive, innovative, and dynamic in a rapidly changing world. In my lifetime I have not seen any issue divide our country as much as health care reform. In some ways I am saddened by this fact. In many ways, however, I recognize that it is healthy for us to dig down deeply and to have this national dialogue in order to uncover issues that have divided our country and polarized so many of our people. If we do not have this public debate and dialogue, these barriers will remain and will continue to trip us up on our path towards better health in America.

The ACA took over one year of intense discussion and debate. It will define the next several generations of health care provision in the United States. Although this bill is not perfect, it is a starting point for at least 20 years of further revision, modification, and improvement. It is a huge step forward for our nation's health care system. It does not matter if you are from a red state or a blue state. It does not matter if you are a Democrat or Republican or liberal, conservative, or independent. It does not matter if you are a man or a woman, rich or poor, young or old. The issue of reforming our health care system is an American issue. It is an economic issue. It is a quality issue. It is a moral issue. It will take time and patience but we will get there. One thing is for sure, we cannot afford to *not* do this.

Chapter 10

THE PATH TO HEALING OUR FRACTURED HEALTH CARE SYSTEM

Winston Churchill said, "America will always do the right thing, after it tries every other option." We must not lose sight of what we're trying to accomplish: a better health care system for all Americans. We need a system that provides basic coverage for all with access to the right physicians and health care teams, at the right time, right locations, and for the right reasons. We want a health care system that is affordable for individuals and families and also for businesses, states, and our nation. We want to bring down health care costs by focusing more on wellness and prevention, instead of paying exorbitant amounts of money only after people are sick or injured. We must build a health care system, not a sick care system, and not a wealth care system.

Now that the largest health care reform law since 1965 has been passed, our nation stands at the first day of the rest of its life. By no means was the passage of the Affordable Care Act an end point. Many have worked hard to turn this bill into law and they must be thanked, but this is just a starting point. We must continue the dialogue to define the right balance, speed, cost, and direction for health care reform. This is critical for our nation. Health care affects every one of us sooner or later and in many complex ways. We each need to contribute our own unique perspective on how to make the best improvements possible. We must diligently work to shape and refine our new health care law into it what it needs to be for the good of all Americans.

With the passage of the Affordable Care Act, we have moved out of the legislative phase into the regulatory phase, and we must now implement the new law's provisions. This will be a long journey. It is like drawing up blueprints for a new building. These blueprints were passed into law, but now we must construct the actual building. To do this we must have money, along with contractors and subcontractors working together with architects and general managers. This will take time; time to get the team working together and time to build it right. We will make mistakes in construction. We will need to change some of the plans. But build we must! I remain optimistic that we will progressively move our health care system in the right direction. We will construct the basic provisions of enhanced coverage, better access, a more balanced health care workforce, much-needed health insurance reform, higher quality, a larger focus on prevention, and lower cost. I believe our great nation is up to this task.

For all the reasons discussed in this book, resistance to change in health care was quite predictable, but the resulting rancor and discord only reinforced why we needed to begin the process. Clearly, at this time it would have been too disruptive and too costly to have delivered even larger reform measures. For reform of this magnitude to America's largest economic sector, initial changes needed to be somewhat incremental. I'm sure there are many who would have preferred more. There are also many who would have preferred less. There are even many who would have preferred no changes at all. The reality is that up front there would not have been buy-in from enough people for a total reform to occur. It was a major stretch to get everyone at the table and talking long enough to forge into law a very difficult health care reform bill.

What we must accomplish going forward is a uniquely American solution. We cannot adopt another country's health care model and expect it to work, given our unique American culture. An American solution to the problem will be by definition a pluralistic system constructed by many different entities, each with a say about health care reform. That is as it should be. However, we must have overarching, aligning principles that help guarantee coverage, access, quality, and cost control. There is no way at this point in American history that a single-payer, government-run system is going to happen. There is just too much mistrust of our federal government, even though nearly 100 million Americans are already covered by a single-payer health care system. Do not forget: Medicare, Medicaid, SCHIP, the Department of Defense Health Care System, the Veterans Affairs Health Care System, and the Indian Health Service now cover approximately one-third of all Americans.

This isn't to imply that a single-payer national system won't emerge down the road; but at this moment in its history, America is not sympathetic with this concept. In fact, if you are a fan of a single-payer, government-run system, you should want to see the Affordable Care Act fail, so that the next iteration takes an even more radical approach, leading perhaps to a federally run, single-payer system. This is because our health care system would be so fractured by that time that there would be demand for even more massive reform, which may or may not be good for our country. On the other hand, since other countries' health care reform models are also works in progress, careful and ongoing scrutiny on how they are reforming health care (using their different models) will be instructive to our own reform journey.

If America's current attempt at health care reform fails, I do not believe we will see another Democratic president achieve success on this in our lifetimes. It would be too politically risky. Too much political capital, time, energy, and resources would be expended to watch it once again fall on the rocks of entrenched forces and special interests. That is not to say that health care reform could not happen, but I believe that it might actually then occur with a Republican president who could inspire the nation, along with receptive Democrats on the other side of the aisle, to extend open hands for the common good. As I have said before, health care reform is not a Democratic or a Republican issue. It is an American issue. It does not reflect Republican values or Democratic values or Independent values but American values.

We must be patient and not have undue expectations of hasty success. Health care reform will not happen overnight, and our nation's health care may well get worse before it gets better. As we expand coverage to 32 million more Americans from 2014 to 2016, we will struggle to provide access to primary care physicians and team-based primary care practices. We will have pent-up demand waiting to receive patient-centered personal physician care; one focused on wellness, prevention, and chronic disease management. Because of the inadequate number of primary care physicians and other primary care providers, we will see increased emergency room utilization and increased total health care cost until the workforce issue can be corrected. Our nation must start immediately to rebuild its decimated primary care workforce and put more of the right types of physicians into position to provide the type of health care reform that we've talked about in this book. That will take time, but those are the correct steps to start taking now.

As we launch our nation's new health care reform law, we must also consider larger forces, not only in our nation, but in the world around us. We are going from the Industrial into the Information Age, which is transforming everything around us. The economic turmoil felt by our nation and the rest of the world is being driven deeply by this electronic Information Age, with the Internet and complex computer systems transforming how life is conducted. Productivity is increasing as we use the Information Age to transform business and all facets of our life including health care. New forces will come into play that will increase competition for business and speed up transactions significantly. This will lead to an increase in uncertainty, fear, and change for change's sake. Those that control information and knowledge will be powerful.

There will be other power changes, not only among nations, but also among generations and gender. Much of America's focus has always been on the young, bold, and dynamic. Emerging will be a shift to our older citizens. This will occur not only because there will be more and more aged Americans, but also because they will become politically more powerful and have the resources, money and Information Age tools to shape change. This will play out in our health care system, pushing it from a free-for-all, unregulated, highly unstable system, catering mostly to those who have insurance or the financial wherewithal, to a much more stable and secure health care system that will act as a safety net for the good of the whole. Women will also play increasingly more important roles in government, business, and health care. This gender shift will bring a broader and more compassionate view, more targeted on ensuring that an accessible, high-quality and efficient health care system is put into place for our nation.

Therefore, as we stand on the verge of the future, what key items must we keep our eye focused on to ensure that America stays on the right health care reform path? I would like to cluster these items into three "must do" priorities followed by a single pivotal question. These three priorities are:

Priority 1: Create a More Healthy America

Priority 2: Structure the Health Care System to Succeed

Priority 3: Pay for Health Care Wisely

THE PIVOTAL QUESTION: WHO CAN MAKE THESE PRIORITIES HAPPEN?

Priority 1: Create a More Healthy America
Focus on Health

America must become a healthier nation. Much of this will come from the front end of health care as we focus more on wellness, health promotion, prevention, and chronic disease management. As I have repeatedly emphasized, appropriate diet, nutrition, exercise, smoking cessation, alcohol reduction, substance abuse reduction, safe sexual practices, stress reduction, driving slower, using seat belts, immunizations, and other behaviors must be made paramount for the health of our nation. We must focus on health and not sickness. We must focus on function and not illness. We must focus on maximizing everyone's potential through good health and not on managing their disease and illness on the back end of failed and missed opportunities for prevention and wellness. These are not easy things to do and will start with attitudinal changes in our nation's psyche and culture, as well as in our personal lives. Let's face it, healthier people cost less than sick people.

Expanded Coverage

All Americans must have health insurance coverage. This is critical. If everyone does not have basic health insurance, then you cannot spread the risk and cost to the population as a whole. Providing coverage to everyone stops such discriminatory health care insurance practices as rescission, insurance denials for preexisting conditions, and other equally egregious health care insurance practices. Having everyone covered allows them access to timely primary care and more focus on wellness and prevention. It allows people to live healthier and longer. It allows people peace of mind.

There must be a basic benefits package that covers wellness, prevention, primary care, mental health care, chronic disease management, vaccinations, and preventive screens. It must also provide catastrophic care on the back end of health care for individuals that need this. We must provide stability and security to people's lives so that they do not become bankrupt if they have a major accident or illness. Providing the front end, basic benefit package to health care will keep people functional, independent, productive, and healthy. This pays off to the nation as a whole by lowering health care costs, maximizing workforce productivity, and allowing the nation to reach its full potential. There are only two actions that have been shown to both increase quality of health care and decrease cost:

1. Ensure that everybody has some type of health insurance.

2. Ensure that everybody has a personal physician and a consistent place where they are cared for (1).

Quality Care

We must relentlessly improve quality in our health care system. We must reduce our medical error rate and continuously practice performance improvement and quality assurance to ensure patient safety. Many who have access to health care do get extraordinarily good care. Our subspecialist and primary care physicians are among the best in the world. The problem is that not enough people have access to these providers. This creates large gaps in our health care system, resulting in poor quality when compared against much of the world. These "disparity gaps" are widening into "disparity graves," leading to an estimated 45,000 premature American deaths a year (2). All people need health care coverage so we can reduce such glaring differences in health care outcomes based on ethnicity, socioeconomics, and whether one has insurance or not. Additionally, for those patients that do have access to health care, there is much waste, inefficiency, and redundancy in the system. Up to one-third of health care costs fall into these categories. To get to a better-performing, higher-quality health care system, we must stop the fragmentation of care. This can be best achieved by comprehensive, continuous-relationship-based primary care in conjunction with integrated health information systems.

Electronic medical records and high-speed information systems should integrate data and communicate it widely. Offices, whether 100 yards or 5,000 miles apart, should be able to communicate as effectively as I can now with my bank at any ATM machine in the world. Health care information should be easily portable anywhere in the world, just like my bank account. The poor communication that happens between clinicians' offices, the emergency room, hospitals, pharmacies, and other providers must improve so that patients are not harmed in the process of getting health care. The Institute of Medicine (IOM) states that as many as 98,000 people die each year in hospitals from preventable errors (3). These needless deaths that occur each year in the United States due to medical error must stop. This is equivalent to losing a Boeing 767 full of passengers each day! Can you imagine what the Federal Aviation Administration and our nation would do to the airline industry if there was a daily crash of a large airliner in the United States? We need to pay better attention to interoperable communication systems, to point-of-service, evidence-based clinical care guidelines, and to engaged patients who are more knowledgeable of their own personal health records. Information needs to flow freely and quickly to help everyone move toward these better-quality outcomes. This is what leveraging health information technology inside the profession of medicine will do.

Repair Health Care Disparities

There must be strong efforts made to decrease the health care disparities that exist among ethnic, racial, and socioeconomic groups. The disparities that exist in mortality and morbidity with cancer, heart disease, heart failure, and diabetes must be more equitably handled. We cannot stand by and watch as one of our countryman dies because of lack of access to health care for something that can be treated. Martin Luther King Jr. once said, "Of all the forms of inequality, the inequality of not having adequate health care is perhaps the most cruel and inhumane." (4)

America must educate more health care providers, physicians, nurses, PAs, and nurse practitioners from broad ethnic and racial backgrounds to help care for these same groups and others as well. As I discussed earlier in this book, the relationship you have with your physician is important to your health. It is through that relationship that health care is leveraged. Having a trusted personal physician who understands your culture, language, traditions, and values should be a goal of our health care system. As noted earlier, the fundamental question becomes: is health care a fundamental right or not? I believe strongly that it is. Therefore, we must redouble our efforts as a country to stop health care discrimination at all levels. Ensuring that people have some form of coverage and a usual place of care will, more than anything else, start to end health care disparities. We owe our nation nothing less than our collective best efforts in this regard.

Priority 2: Structure the Health Care System to Succeed
Primary Care

The place for people to achieve a trusting relationship with high-quality personal care is with a primary care physician and his or her team. These are family physicians, general internists, general pediatricians, and geriatricians, who can provide a new model of care: the patient-centered medical home, a concept that America is now beginning to use to reorient our health care system around patient-centeredness. Perhaps a more appropriate term would have been "person"-centered medical home. The use of "person" versus "patient" reflects a more proactive, empowered, holistic approach. It focuses more on the health of the individual than on a dependent, reactive sick care approach, implied by the term "patient." For the sake of this writing, however, I will use the term patient-centered medical home, as this is the term more generally accepted.

The patient-centered medical home is not only a place (i.e., a practice location) where patients receive integrated and coordinated care, but is also a care process that is delivered through an expanded team of providers using electronic medical records and information technology to coordinate comprehensive, continuous health care. Again, it is patient-centered, meaning that it is the patient, as an engaged active participant, who is in charge of their care. The physician and his or her extended team are partners with the patient and share in the responsibility of creating a health care plan that meets the patient's needs, desires, and goals. If there is no basic interface with the health care system through a personal physician who knows the patient and his or her family and their community, there can be no trusted, informed assessment of what is best for the individual patient's health. Everything in the health care system should work around this interface (See Figure 1).

Figure 1. The Patient–Physician Relationship

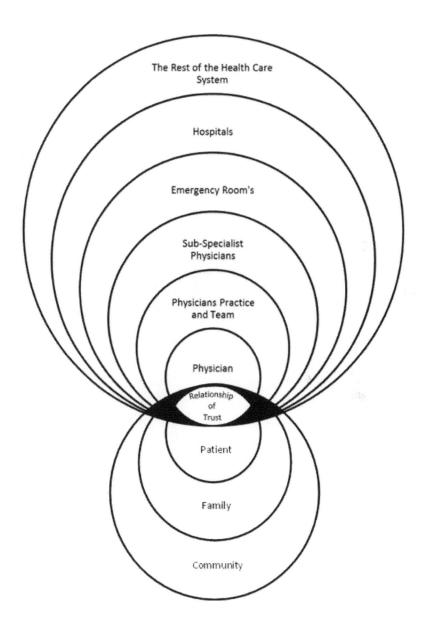

Studies, as pointed out earlier in the book, have shown both the increased quality and increased satisfaction of this approach. Morbidity and mortality are reduced and value as defined as quality divided by cost is greatly enhanced (5).

Figure 2 illustrates the concept of the patient-centered medical home, structured around a patient-centered, physician-directed starting point. On this it builds a core foundation of family medicine and primary care, with its comprehensive, continuous, and relationship-based components. The patient-centered medical home then introduces a culture of improvement using quality metrics, such as performance measurement and reliable information collection systems, to better provide patients what they need. It then adds the patient's satisfaction, measured by convenient access to coordinated and personalized care, followed by efficient practice organization in the form of financial management, personnel management, and clinical systems. Finally it adds effective health information technology, including business and clinical process automation, information connectivity and communication, evidence-based medicine support, and clinical data analysis and representation. All of these layers of the patient-centered medical home are used to provide great outcomes. If you will, it is like having Dr. Marcus Welby in the Information Age. These outcomes are good for patients who enjoy better health and share in health care decisions. They are good for physicians who can now focus on delivering excellent medical care. They are good for practices, allowing the team to work together effectively, with the resources needed to support excellent patient care. They are also good for payers and employers in that they drive quality and efficiency, and avoid unnecessary costs.

Figure 2. The Patient-Centered Medical Home

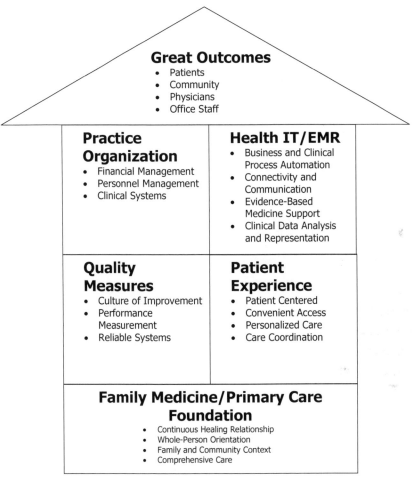

Great Outcomes
- Patients
- Community
- Physicians
- Office Staff

Practice Organization
- Financial Management
- Personnel Management
- Clinical Systems

Health IT/EMR
- Business and Clinical Process Automation
- Connectivity and Communication
- Evidence-Based Medicine Support
- Clinical Data Analysis and Representation

Quality Measures
- Culture of Improvement
- Performance Measurement
- Reliable Systems

Patient Experience
- Patient Centered
- Convenient Access
- Personalized Care
- Care Coordination

Family Medicine/Primary Care Foundation
- Continuous Healing Relationship
- Whole-Person Orientation
- Family and Community Context
- Comprehensive Care

Patient Centered | Physician Directed

Source: Modified from the American Academy of Family Physicians—The Patient-Centered Medical Home. April 2009 (6)

To have the right types of physicians and other providers deliver health care in the patient-centered medical home, every effort should be made to rapidly expand the primary care workforce. The system is in great imbalance now with only 30 percent of the workforce being in primary care, a percentage that is dropping rapidly. The Council on Graduate Medical Education (COGME) in its 20th Annual Report is calling for at least 40 percent of the nation's workforce to be in primary care (7). This is the minimum number of primary care physicians we must have in our country. A goal to shoot for will be to have 50 percent of the workforce in primary care (like most of the industrialized countries of the world).

To achieve this goal, there must be payment reform that values what primary care physicians do and works on a blended payment system consisting of four parts:

1. An enhanced fee-for-service for face-to-face visits.

2. A care management fee for non-face-to-face service time (i.e., telephone calls, e-mail visits, coordination of care with other subspecialists in the medical home "neighborhood").

3. Quality incentives for maximizing patient outcomes (i.e., getting blood pressure and diabetes controlled, getting immunization rates for children and adults above certain percentages, etc.).

4. A shared savings component in which financial savings from decreased emergency room visits, hospitalizations, and high cost pharmacy overutilization are shared with the practices and their patients as incentives to better health oriented outcomes.

This will move us away from a quantity-driven, fee-for-service dominated system to one based on high-value and quality outcomes. It will help the primary care physician get off the hamster treadmill in the current fee-for-service model of trying to cover overhead by seeing more and more patients. Instead it gives the physician the freedom to deliver care in a more relaxed atmosphere where he or she does not need to see high volumes of patients to be successful. In the patient-centered medical home much of the patient's care can be handled by the primary care physician and other team members by email, telephone, and other information technology sources that provide asynchronous, non-face-to-face interactions allowing questions, answers, and information sharing that are paid for and valued. In essence, it moves us from a volume-based health care system to a value-based health care system.

For all of this to function efficiently, there must be a strong relationship between health care providers and the patient. Let me describe a vision of what this health care system of tomorrow might look like in the primary care physician's office. Instead of seeing 20 to 50 patients a day in face-to-face visits, the family physician of tomorrow will see eight to 12 patients a day, four to six in the morning and four to six in the afternoon. How can this be possible, you are probably thinking? How can those who see family physicians and other primary care physicians only amount to eight to 12 patients a day? The answer is, because they are healthier and don't need to be seen so frequently, and their ongoing health care needs will often be met in ways other than taking the time and expense to be seen directly in the primary care physician's office. A sign of an effective and efficient primary care practice will be to have an empty waiting room, not a full one. Why? Because the patients will be having their health care needs met in non-face-to-face visits: by telephone, by e-mail, by interactive websites and patient education tools. What will be happening in asynchronous, non-face-to-face visits? There will be 10 to 30 e-mails or phone calls that the primary care physicians and his/her expanded team will handle in the morning, another 10 to 20 at lunch time, and another 10 to 30 at the end of the day. Reports on lab results, x-rays, and consultations with other health care providers will happen then. Follow-up on chronic diseases such as diabetes, asthma, emphysema, heart failure, depression, cancer, hypertension, and other chronic diseases can be handled through new mechanisms of information technology in proactive, health-achieving ways. Questions about new symptoms or problems can be raised and handled electronically or telephonically. Needs can be anticipated and demands can be handled. Proactive educational resources with interactive video messaging and algorithm-directed questions can occur that lead to answers and deeper understanding and engagement of a patient with their disease.

All of this of course will be paid for in reasonable ways. A reasonable charge for an e-mail or telephone call will help pay the primary care physician and their team for their expertise and time, and will save the patient time during a busy day from needing to see the physician. The insurance companies will save money by paying less for these virtual visits than for face-to-face visits. This is a win-win-win. It is a win for the patient to be kept proactively healthy and not just treated reactively when sick. It is a win for the primary care physician to be valued, respected, and paid for their team's expertise, and to manage the health-related issues of all of their patients in a timely way, preventing physician stress and burn out. It will also be a win for the insurance companies and the health care industry to become more efficient and reduce the cost of health care. By providing this patient-centered, proactive care there will be reduced emergency room visits, hospitalizations, and overall cost of medical care. If you think this is impossible, then think again. This benefit is already being seen all across the nation in demonstration pilots from North Carolina, to Pennsylvania, to Washington, to Minnesota, to Colorado, to Utah, to Maryland (8, 9, 10, 11, 12, 13, 14). In fact, these early patient-centered medical home pilots are showing decreased emergency room utilization of 15 to 50 percent, decreased hospitalization rates of 10 to 40 percent, and decreased cost per patient of approximately $835 per patient per year (8, 9, 10, 11, 12, 13, 14).

Now what about those four to six patients in the morning and four to six patients in the afternoon? They are patients who truly need to be seen, and need to have the physician and his/her team spend time caring for them in a relaxed, non-hurried way that provides high-quality care. They can be those patients with multiple medical problems that you just need extra time with, or patients that have a mental health problem in conjunction with a chronic medical disease who may take a bit longer to untangle the important questions they have. This also provides time to see a patient with an acute same-day problem that could not be handled by your team by a phone call or email. It could also provide time for the complex patient that needs the primary care physician's skills, in addition to those of the team, to sort through several preventive and intense education needs associated with behavior change and wellness which will make big health care changes down the road. Now that is a vision of future health care that I know my primary care colleagues want to see. It gets us all off of the proverbial hamster treadmill of reactive sick care and focuses instead on proactive, timely, quality health care.

There must also be enhanced loan repayment and scholarships for those who choose to go into primary care so that we can rearm our workforce with outstanding, high-quality primary care physicians who will serve the public and build a relationship of trust that will be the basis for the patient-centered medical home. Along with these changes, America's medical schools must transform their training model to focus more on producing community-based primary care physicians. We must get away from the model that currently exists in the American medical school system that overstresses the production of a subspecialty workforce that's good for teaching hospitals, academic health centers, and research labs. Without question we must have subspecialists and researchers produced by medical schools, but there needs to better balance given and greater attention paid to the needs of the community-based primary care workforce.

As a nation we must produce a symphony of care. This symphony of care is similar to a musical symphony. We must have a balance of woodwinds, brass, strings, and percussion. To produce the most beautiful sound possible it must play in harmony. It must be balanced. Right now the American health care system is out of balance. It has too many subspecialists. It would be like our symphony orchestra having too many tubas and not enough violins. Our health care symphony is not playing beautiful music because of this asymmetry. Continuing this analogy, a symphony also needs a conductor: someone who has a broad vision of how the parts of the symphony must play together, one who integrates, one who coordinates. It needs someone who connects the dots into a synergistic whole. The indispensible conductor in our analogous health care symphony is the primary care physician. It is the primary care physician who has the broad vision of the health care system, who knows how best to deploy the rest of the team in providing the right type of care by the right health care provider in the right health care setting. The primary care physician's role as the conductor of the health care symphony team is critical for timely, accessible, quality, and affordable care. Without a strong primary-care-based system all you have is a jumble of independent instruments not playing together well and not producing the beautiful music that all of them are capable of performing. As I've stated earlier: we must get at least 40 percent of the workforce in primary care as soon as possible, and we cannot rest until that number gets to 50 percent if we truly want our health care system to maximize its full potential as an accessible, affordable, and high-quality health care symphony.

In order to increase the primary care physician workforce now, not only must there be attention on increasing the pipeline of primary care physicians on the front end through medical schools, but we also must slow down the retirement of primary care physicians on the back end of this pipeline. These experienced physicians have shouldered the great responsibility of taking care of their patients through this time of a broken health care system. They must be acknowledged and thanked for their outstanding work. There must also be attention paid and incentives given to help these physicians find the energy and effort to continue to practice while we work hard to balance America's health care workforce.

These primary care physicians have worked long and hard, and have been frustrated by a system that systematically undervalues their skills and has underpaid them for what they bring to health care and their individual patients. Many have borne the brunt of the administrative burden and paperwork that disproportionately targets primary care physicians. In a recent study, 73.4 items are brought to the average primary care physician per day are not paid for. These comprise 16.8 e-mails per day, 12.1 prescription refills per day, 19.5 laboratory reports per day, 11.1 imaging reports per day, and 13.9 consultation reports per day (15). Additionally, 52 minutes each day are spent on extra administrative paperwork by each primary care physician. This represents an extra 4.3 hours each week that is lost to paperwork instead of seeing patients (16). Not only are the physicians spending this extra time, but so are their staffs. Nursing staff is spending 14 hours and clerical staff is spending 45 hours per week on these extra duties (16). Many have labored long and hard, and are quite frankly burned out with medicine. This has led to an absolute crisis in primary care. At the exact time that we are talking about expanding coverage to more of America's citizens and at a time when our Medicare population will be doubling from 40 to 80 million people in the next 15 years, we are losing our primary care workforce. How contradictory is it that as we try to solve America's health care crisis, we are under-producing the exact types of physicians that can fix the problem. Conversely, we are over-producing the wrong types of physicians (i.e., the subspecialists) who cannot fix the problem. The nation as a whole must work hard to attract and reward primary care physicians for the value they bring to the health care system.

Once we get our health care system re-centered on primary care, and working more efficiently, the citizens of our states will keep it in place. The reason is that 95 percent of the patients will then be getting access to ongoing high-quality, accessible, and timely care through their own primary care physicians. This high-quality care will be very satisfying to the patient through a personal, trusted relationship. If our elected representatives cannot ensure that this type of health care system then continues to exist for their citizens, they will be voted out of office. In other words, once the shift occurs and this type of health care system goes into place, it will be the people themselves who will continue to hold on to it. This is how it has happened in other industrialized countries in the world (17). It is time for this to happen in America as well. In *The Omnivore's Dilemma*, Michael Pollan writes, "Eat food, not too much, mostly plants." (18) A similar quote was penned by one of my colleagues, Kevin Grumbach, a family physician, at the University of California, San Francisco, "Get health care, not too much, mostly primary care."

Community Care Versus Hospital Care

An emerging trend in health care is a movement away from hospitals and into the communities. Hospitals will always be needed for certain types of care, but we now rely on them disproportionately at the back end of downstream health care as opposed to focusing proactively on front-end care of upstream health care in community offices of primary care physicians and other community services. This has set up an expensive, reactive health care system where procedures, imaging, and "things" are done to patients, as contrasted to the proactive system of primary health care and patient education in an ambulatory environment where things are prevented from needing to be done to patients. As health care reform moves forward, the pendulum must swing more towards cost effective, higher quality, preventive, outpatient settings and less toward the back end of medicine with expensive, overpriced hospitalizations and emergency rooms. The figure in Chapter 1 demonstrates what happens to a thousand patients over the course of a month. Most don't need to go to emergency rooms and hospitals. If we begin to focus more of our health care efforts and dollars in community settings, then health will happen and costs will be greatly reduced. That should be our nation's goal. We will know we have become successful when we start to reduce ER visits and hospitalizations per capita, and when all Americans have timely access to high-quality primary care, diminished disparities in care along racial and ethnic lines, and longer life spans.

On a related topic, emergency rooms and hospitals should be utilized by the right patients, at the right time, for the right reasons and not because there's a lack of access to appropriate primary care. A patient defaulting to an emergency room through lack of access to a primary care physician is a symptom of our fractured health care system. It is a symptom of our nation's health care disease. That disease is the lack of primary care access. Emergency rooms should be for true medical emergencies. Emergency rooms and emergency medicine is attractive and exciting on TV dramas, but primary care in community offices is where the majority of health care in our country takes place. It will be even more so in the future. We cannot fail to get this right as we "re-form" our health care system.

Nurse Practitioners and Physician Assistants

There must be enhanced collaboration and partnering between primary care physicians, nurse practitioners, and physician assistants. Quite frankly, there will not be enough primary care physicians in the next 10 years to meet the growing demand as we refocus health care delivery to the front end of medicine while expanding health care coverage to 32 million more Americans. There must be more nurse practitioners and physician assistants who work in harmony with primary care physicians to coordinate, integrate, and organize health care using their talents under the team leadership of primary care physicians. This is consistent with the whole concept of the patient-centered medical home team. Even in those states where nurse practitioners can legally practice independently, without physician oversight, they should still work in concert with primary care physicians in an organized way so as to not overwhelm the consultants in the subspecialty arenas with consultations that could be best handled in the primary care arena.

If there is not collaboration and partnering with primary care physicians in a team oriented fashion, the difference in the scope of practice between nurse practitioners, physician assistants, and primary care physicians can result in overutilization of health care. One troubling trend in both the nurse practitioner (NP) and physician assistant (PA) communities is of subspecialization. Both groups are doing exactly what is being done by physicians, and for the same reasons. They are following the money. Both the NP and PA professions came into existence to provide more primary care help. But subspecialization trends have impacted them greatly with only 52 percent of NPs now doing primary care and only 43 percent of PAs still doing primary care (19). The incentives under the current system are not aligned to produce primary care physicians and providers. That must change going forward to "re-form" and re-balance the health care workforce. Primary care must be a team sport. The mantra going forward, as shared with me by a wonderful Canadian family physician colleague of mine named Cal Gutkin, should be that every patient in America "deserves a physician *and* a nurse"; a physician *and* a nurse practitioner or physician assistant. The message going forward should not be that every patient should have a "physician *or* a nurse"; a "physician *or* a nurse practitioner *or* physician assistant." The concept of a team is to synergistically use each other's skills to achieve higher performance, not to divide the team into piecemeal parts that reduces performance, quality, outcomes, and cost. This will be an ongoing challenge for physicians, NPs, and PAs, but I believe the leadership abilities of all three of these important provider groups can work together for the good of health care and patients of our nation. There is enough work for all of us to do. It will be more effectively done if we do it together.

Electronic Medical Records (EMRs) and Health Information Technology (HIT)

As we move into the Information Age, medicine has yet to escape from the Industrial Age, where, because of its payment structure, it has been mired. Clinging to the status quo of existing systems has been more of the norm than the exception, even though avant-garde practices using electronic medical records and information technology have been around for 20 years. Why is it then that most physicians' offices and hospitals in the United States are not using electronic medical records? A lot has to do with cost. In many medical offices across the country margins are thin and there are no payment incentives to adopt this new technology. Incentives are needed to encourage the use of electronic medical records and high-speed health information technology by physicians, emergency rooms, hospitals, and other health care providers. This should be simple, seamless, interoperable, and geared to the patient's needs. You would think that this would be a no-brainer for the profession of medicine in America, but it has been a real struggle. EMR and HIT adoption has lagged behind other industrialized nations and we have struggled to get up to speed in this important arena. That is why the American Recovery and Reinvestment Act (ARRA), also known as the stimulus bill, set aside $19 billion for EMR and HIT adoption by physicians, hospitals, and health care systems, as a down-payment to jump-start this journey. Remember that America's physicians, practices, health care systems, and hospitals have been slow to do this because the cost came right out of their pockets. In other industries, such as the retail industry, these costs can be passed on to the customer. This is not true in medicine, where payments are predefined by contracts and fixed payment and cannot be arbitrarily increased and passed on to patients, insurance companies, or the federal government.

All medical schools and residency programs must ensure that medical students and residents are well trained to use electronic medical records and handheld computing devices to bring information to the patient's bedside or their physician's office. These electronic systems pull together information in legible and readable formats. They help alert health care teams to dangerous lab values or x-ray findings. They help avoid medication errors such as wrong doses or interactions that may occur between different medications (or between a patient's medical condition and a certain medication that could make that condition worse). It will help identify a medication that should not be given because the patient has a known allergy to that medication. Electronic medical records and information systems can also help avoid redundancy and duplication of tests and studies, saving patients unnecessary and expensive tests. Perhaps the single greatest advantage will be to have as much accurate medical information as is possible present so the best medical decisions can be made for the patient. It is time for the profession of medicine to move into the Information Age.

Priority 3: Pay for Health Care Wisely
Health Creation Versus Wealth Creation

Just as there must be a better balance under health care reform between resources devoted to primary versus specialty care, there must be a shift in balance to identify health care as being the ultimate end point, rather than simply as a way to create wealth. This is an important distinction. The goal of health care should be to produce health for the people of our country and should not be to produce wealth for entities such as hospitals, physicians, health insurance companies, stockholders, pharmaceutical companies, and medical device manufacturers. Therefore, incentives must be aligned to move our nation towards better health care, and at the same time to control costs and put discipline in wealth generation. The two can coexist. It's not an either/or proposition, but the creation of health must be the higher priority. After all, medicine should be much more about being a profession and less about being a business.

Health Insurance Reform

Much overdue effort has been expended in the health care reform law to reform health insurance. It is important to provide people some form of health insurance coverage, but we must stop health insurance abuses and discrimination that can actually harm people. The Affordable Care Act takes significant steps in the right direction. Just to mention a few: no longer will there be denials for preexisting conditions; nonrenewals based on illness, sickness, or injury; caps placed on out-of-pocket expenses; rescissions for becoming sick; or gender discrimination. Health insurance should exist solely to help people pay for their health care and their health. It should be a bridge and not a barrier. It should be about patients and families. Health insurance should be seen as their friend and not their enemy. It should be the paying part of health care, not just part of the system of wealth generation for the health insurance sector, its CEOs and leaders, and stockholders. The ability to produce a common set of guidelines and standards that are transparent will be helpful to everyone. So too will administrative simplification so that the paperwork does not overwhelm the providers or the patients. No longer should there be monumentally slow payments from health insurance companies so that they can generate additional revenue through interest on money they should be paying in timely ways to physicians, hospitals, and other health care entities. Simple, clear health insurance policies and programs using understandable language and offered in the one-stop shopping health exchanges will be helpful for both individuals and businesses. These simplified and standardized rules will decrease confusion and produce exactly what health insurance is designed for: providing health care coverage and payment on behalf of patients so that they can maximize their health and minimize their sickness, disease, and injuries.

People most need their health insurance when they become ill, but the way the system has operated, insurance companies could drop you because you *have* become ill. Provisions in the health care reform bill will ensure that insurance companies are prohibited from dropping or decreasing an individual's coverage, or markedly increasing a patient's premium, when they become sick. As has been stated throughout this book, America's health care system must focus on the front end of health care. It is frustrating that insurance companies have often not paid for care that would prevent more expensive payouts downstream and have not paid for problems that could have been prevented or favorably modified in the first place. Finally, under these provisions, insurance companies must fully cover you for regular check-ups and preventive exams. All of these changes are about "re-forming" the health care system.

Cost Control

Cost is the specter that haunts health reform in our nation (2). There must be relentless effort to bring down this cost. Again, America's health care is twice as expensive as the average for the rest of the industrialized countries and 40 percent higher than the next closest country (20). It would perhaps be worth that if our health care outcomes were at least double the average of the rest of the world's industrialized nations or 40 percent higher than the next closest country, but we only have mediocre health care outcomes from this excessive spending (21). In fact, we rank 19th out of 19 countries on a measure of mortality amenable to medical care and have fallen from 15th on this measure over the last several years (22). What this means is that even though we spend by far the most on health care of any country on Earth, we rank last in the industrialized countries (19 of 19) in deaths that might have been prevented with timely and effective care.

We have overpriced health care in our country, and overvalued procedures and imaging. This cost will need to come down as we shift dollars to the front end of health care with prevention, chronic disease management, and health care promotion. Independent panels of experts made up of both public and private individuals, using consumers and primary care physicians, must help evaluate the costs of our health care system. In the new Affordable Care Act, the Independent Payment Advisory Board (IPAB) will serve in this role. It will need to use the best evidence, knowledge and judgment to critically and fairly reevaluate the cost of procedures, services, and imaging. Most likely there will be multiple sources of knowledge and data to help with this decision-making. This is not rationing. This is the intelligent utilization of data-based decision-making to correct a capsized health care system. It will address questions such as: how can it be that the same MRI of the brain costs $105 in Japan and $1400 in the United States? (23)

Tough decisions need to be made when managing cost. That is why evidence determining what care works effectively will need to be used to make the best possible decisions on how to achieve the best clinical outcomes. This isn't the denial of care; it is the selection of the best possible care using informed evidence. That choice must be shared between the physician and the patient based on this evidence and based on value. The highest value is obtained when you have high quality and low cost. The lowest value is obtained when you have low quality and high cost. Would you buy a car without knowing something about its dependability, quality, and cost? So why do we not have open knowledge discussions about these issues for purchasing health care?

Along with cutting expense in the system, there must be increased revenue generated through taxation as well. It will be up to Congress to decide how best to do this, but things that are known to contribute to poor health in our country must be looked at for increased taxation. Just as cigarettes have been a source of revenue through increased taxation, should such items as sugared beverages, cookies, and candy also be taxed? Should there be increased taxation on alcohol? If these items in excess are known to be associated with poor health and increased health care costs, should they be taxed just as cigarettes are? Our nation needs to sort through both the pros and cons of these decisions. Similarly, other creative areas in which external revenue can be raised and plowed back into a first-rate, outstanding health care system should be thought through. We must try to do this in a balanced way so that we are not asking our citizens to pay more taxes across the board, but to look more towards taxation on items that can actually harm health and help deter excessive use.

As the number of patients in Medicare doubles over the next 15 years, perhaps it is time to look at means-testing for Medicare patients. Many elderly Americans have become very successful financially through their lives. Good for them. I'm sure they have certainly earned that. However, should there be some appropriate scaling of what they need to pay to have Medicare health insurance as opposed to those that live paycheck to paycheck on Social Security or disability payments? As we go forward, I submit that we need to take a long, hard, and careful look at how we structure Medicare insurance payments from the patient side. This should not penalize people, but provide a more level playing field based on their wealth and income. I'm sure this suggestion will not make some people happy, but it is the right thing to do in an effort to help control cost so as many people as possible can get adequately covered. Again, the needs of the many must outweigh the needs of the few.

Liability Reform

The fact that liability reform was not more of a central focus of our health care reform debate speaks for the stranglehold that the legal profession and trial lawyers have as a special interest and lobbying activity, as well as the impact they have on Congress. This is a glaring deficit in our health care reform bill, despite the fact that some positive steps were taken in terms of grants for states to look at more innovative ways of resolving disputes over medical liability. As I witnessed up close and personal over these last seven years of health care reform, the one group of people that was not around the table were the trial attorneys and malpractice lawyers. They deftly avoided what should have amounted to major reform in the liability system. It has been estimated that the cost of liability premiums alone are $26 billion annually, which represents a 2,000 percent increase since 1975 (24). This represents a 12 percent growth annually in premium rates and exceeds the inflation rate by 400 percent and medical spending rate increases by 200 percent (25). Million dollar settlements are now the norm with 52 percent of awards exceeding $1 million and the average award being $4.7 million (26). The cost of malpractice in a recent *Health Affairs* article on this topic is approximately $55.6 billion per year, which represents 2.4 percent of all health care spending (27). These concerns and fears have led physicians, especially those without long-standing relationships with patients, to over-order tests, labs, x-rays, and other imaging studies and consultations with subspecialists. These fears of being sued have led to overuse of emergency rooms by physicians who are called after hours by patients, over-hospitalization of patients as opposed to watchful waiting, and doing procedures and surgeries on patients when perhaps they were not needed. A recent Gallup poll revealed 73 to 92 percent of all physicians practice defensive medicine (28). All of this adds up to anywhere in the range of $55.6 billion to $124 billion being spent annually in the practice of defensive medicine (27, 29, 30).

Ongoing health care reform for the good of our nation must look at ways in which we can bring common sense back in to malpractice so that we stop the overwhelming wasteful spending of defensive medicine. When upwards of $124 billion per year is being spent in the practice of defensive medicine, that's money that could be saved by the system and plowed back into better health care. The legal system and medical liability tort reform will see its day in Congress in the near future. It has to if we are truly serious about reforming health care.

PIVOTAL QUESTION: WHO CAN MAKE THESE PRIORITIES HAPPEN?

Simple answer: It is up to the American people to "re-form" our fractured health care system for our country. But this will depend on our collective will.

So what are the next steps for the American people? What are the lessons learned? What do the glimpses into our soul and our character revealed by the health care reform struggle tell us? Who do we see looking back at us when we look into the mirror of health care reform?

One obvious insight is that we are a young nation compared to the rest of the nations in the industrialized world. We are a mere 236 years old; many nations are thousands of years old. In fact, several of our states are just over 100 years old and several are less than 100 years old. We have people in our country older than several of our states. Because of our relative youth and immaturity, we act that way. Instead of stability and security being hallmarks for our nation, we value youth, passion, independence, and choice. These are the struggles of adolescence, and we are an adolescent nation. Many issues in the health care reform debate have centered on how this would affect individuals, not the nation as a whole—more about "me" and less about "us." It became more concerned with those who reaped the benefits of the status quo rather than give up something for the greater good. It became more about self-serving than it did about putting the group or the nation before self.

Our next step as we grow from adolescence into adulthood as a nation is to trade some of our selfishness and independence for security and stability. It is for us as a nation to think more about the whole than the individual. It is for us as a country to act more for the long term good of all than the short-term, shortsighted gain of the individual. Having children teaches this to parents. Our nation will get there, but it will take more time and travail until we do. We are a great nation made up of many good people. We are also a very diverse nation reflecting our immigration history and ancestry. Because our country's birth was based on independence, choice, and autonomy, we have become a nation that does not like being told what to do. Our diversity is our strength, but it is also our weakness. We have become very polarized and distrustful. We have not been able to pull together easily and in fact, the ideological divide is growing. Our effort to achieve health care reform for the good of our nation has become a symptom of our disease. That disease is our basic inability to see that everyone's health care should be his or her own right. No one who desires basic health care should have that basic right denied. It is through the provision of health care to all that we all become stronger, and our nation becomes stronger. That is what we should all strive for.

THE PATH TO HEALING OUR FRACTURED HEALTH CARE SYSTEM

As we work together on our long trek towards a world-class health care system for Americans, what signposts are there along the way that will reassure us that we are progressing in the right direction? In this book I've endeavored to answer this question in considerable detail from multiple viewpoints. The challenge of health care reform is a complex and constantly changing one. But to a hiker on a difficult trail, the best signposts are usually those that are brief and to the point. So, as a final review, here are the key markers we should look for along our path to better health care:

1. **Start with Basic Principles:** We must start with a clear goal. We want our health care system to be accessible, affordable, accountable, and of high quality. We want it to integrate and coordinate care in order to reduce fragmentation and redundancy within the system. We want it to focus on prevention and proactively keeping people healthy. Remember that healthier people cost less than sick people.

2. **Recognize Health Care as a Basic Right**: A fundamental principle for the United States to grapple with as we redesign our health care system is that everyone should be afforded basic health care. This is a basic philosophical premise that our country must reach a consensus on if we intend to repair our current "have" and "have-not" health care system and stop the disparities in care that occur along ethnic and socioeconomic lines. Once we agree on this essential premise, much of the rest of getting our health care system right will fall into place.

3. **Be Person-Centered**: The center of our health care system should be the people we are serving; not the hospitals, the physicians, the insurance companies, the pharmaceutical industry, or others. It should be as people-friendly and user-friendly as possible. If we use the people we are serving as the center of our compass, the right decisions will be made regarding health care.

4. **Be Primary Care-Oriented**: The entire health care system should be rebuilt on a primary care model focused on health

and prevention, not just disease or sickness. Comprehensive, continuous, and integrated care is the change needed to get the United States on the right track. The data is clear that with a primary care-based system, quality, access, and patient satisfaction improve and costs come down. This is the foundational model used in the rest of the world's successful health care systems.

5. **Gather Care Around the Patient-Centered Medical Home (PCMH)**: The beating heart of a redesigned primary care system should be the patient-centered medical home, where an expanded medical team works on behalf of the patient, combining timely, accessible, integrated, and patient-centered care. This ensures accountable, high-quality care focused on the patient and links them to the rest of the health care system when necessary.

6. **Use Health Information Technology (HIT)/Electronic Medical Records (EMR)**: Within the models of primary care and the patient-centered medical home is the integrating tool of the electronic medical record, which allows the PCMH to gather, coordinate, analyze, and share information bi-directionally with practices, patients, and other health care providers (hospitals, ERs, subspecialist physicians). It allows the PCMHs to track patients and clusters of patients with similar problems in efficient and effective ways to proactively maximize their health. Having all of this information stored on a transportable personal "health card" that can immediately upload medical information into the EMR or download that day's medical visit onto the health card should be a goal we strive to achieve.

7. **Provide a Basic Benefit Package**: Built into the Affordable Care Act (ACA) is the basic benefit insurance package. This

package must contain the basic provision of primary care. There must be timely and accessible care from high quality primary care physicians (family physicians, general internal medicine, general pediatricians, and geriatricians). These PCMH-based practices must be accessible to all patients and provide timely acute, chronic, and prevention-based medical care. Further referral can then be coordinated within the rest of the medical system when necessary. These key provisions must be built into the basic insurance package in order to ensure its centrality of function.

8. **Deploy a Balanced Medical Workforce**: To provide enough family physicians/primary care physicians to serve our re-designed system of primary care-based PCMHs, we must have more primary care physicians produced by our nation's medical and osteopathic schools. We now stand at roughly 30 percent of the workforce being in primary care. This ideally must be at 50 percent. This rebuilt primary care workforce will consist of primary care physicians, physician assistants, and nurse practitioners. Medical schools must become more accountable to producing this workforce for the communities' best health outcomes.

9. **Activate the Workforce Commission**: The ACA called for the creation of a national workforce commission to make recommendations to HHS and Congress on the future make-up and distribution of America's health care workforce. These workforce recommendations would affect all professions involved in health care, including physicians, nurses, social workers, psychologists, dentists, and others. This commission had 15 commissioners named, but non-appropriated funding has kept them from meeting. This group needs to meet and make its recommendations so we can intelligently design our future workforce as opposed to reflexively lurching around

and reacting to the free-for-all of our current health care system.

10. **Align Financial Incentives**: The reason our health care system looks and acts the way it does is because financial incentives have built it that way. Follow the money! We must change the financial incentives and realign them to build a quality accessible, patient-centered, and cost-effective health care system. This realignment of financial incentives is a must to achieve the health care system that we will need for our nation's future. This realignment must be heavily toward primary care and health-promoting outcomes.

11. **Use Blended Payment**: We must get away from a total fee-for-service payment structure. This only encourages a volume-driven system based on quantity, not value. The blended payment system includes at least four components: a fee-for-service component for face-to-face visits, a care management fee for non-face-to-face services, a quality component for health care outcomes, and a shared savings component to encourage reductions in cost and utilization of ERs, hospitalizations, and high-priced pharmaceuticals. If the payment mechanisms are redesigned to financially reward the outcomes we seek in our health care system, then those behaviors will happen.

12. **Require Patient Accountability**: For our future health care system to work maximally, patients must take ownership of their health care. They must be accountable as well in a shared partnership with their primary care physicians and their PCMH team-based practices. They must be informed, educated, and made more health literate so that decisions become theirs to make. This will dramatically increase compliance, engagement, and behavior change. This is key to

healthier patient outcomes, better-satisfied patients, and a healthier nation. Patients should also be rewarded for this accountability and health literacy in the form of decreased co-payments and decreased premiums.

13. **Incentivize Healthy Patient Behavior**: If we are going to change the financial incentives for physician, hospital, and health care system behavior we must for patients as well. Appropriate financial incentives to patients for healthy behaviors (smoking cessation, weight loss, exercise) and meeting identified health outcomes (ideal body weight, blood pressure, diabetes management, cholesterol control, and vaccinations) are but a few examples of incentives that will align patients and the system toward health.

14. **Penalize Non-Healthy Patient Behaviors**: Conversely, if patients fail to modify their behavior toward healthier outcomes, they should pay higher premiums or co-pays for their insurance. This would not be designed to limit their ability to obtain insurance but to incentivize movement toward healthier behaviors. Similarly, the nation should impose taxes on products known to be harmful to health. Examples of these would be for tobacco, alcohol, candy, highly sugared beverages, etc.

15. **Expand Coverage**: Once we have the basic tenants of primary care, the PCMH, and the expanded primary care workforce in place, we can expand coverage to everyone in the United States. By having everyone in and no one out, we stop the problem with the uninsured. We stop the disparities in care. We stop people living sicker and dying younger because they cannot access health care. By having people covered with the basic benefit package we start moving them towards the front end of proactive, preventive, and wellness health care

and away from back-end reactive, sickness, and disease care. By having as many people as possible covered we stop the cost shifting of the uninsured on to the premiums of the insured. By having people adequately covered, we stop medical bankruptcies.

16. **Require the Individual Mandate**: An important mechanism in expanding care is to require that everyone has health care insurance and a primary care PCMH to go to for their health care. The individual mandate enables this. Health insurance needs to be reasonably priced with federal subsidies based on income for individuals and families that do not have employer-based insurance. By linking affordable and obtainable health insurance to the individual we assure expanded health insurance coverage and can move all Americans toward the benefits of an integrated and coordinated health care system. Even if the individual mandate is not upheld by the Supreme Court, we must get as many people on some sort of health insurance or health care coverage as possible so that they can be provided timely, accessible health care, where problems are caught early and not reacted to late when costs are higher.

17. **Focus on Prevention**: By getting these systems of care in place, we can truly focus on prevention. We will have the appropriate mind-set of health and health care; we will have the appropriate places (the PCMH) for prevention to be implemented; and we will have the appropriate financial incentives to physicians, practices, and patients to have this become the center piece of our redesigned health care system. The National Prevention Health Promotion and Public Health Council was created in the ACA. This Council needs to be robustly funded and empowered to set priorities and recommendations to HHS and Congress for a healthier America.

18. **Set Quality Benchmarks**: The ACA called for a National Quality Improvement Strategy. This must exist at all levels of the health care system from outpatient practices, to inpatient hospital standards, to public health standards. This strategy would set priorities on health care services delivery, health care outcomes, population health, and the creation and usage of quality measures. Authorizing an expert commission to develop these standards will define goals that the health care system can align towards and be rewarded (or penalized) depending on goal attainment. If you want quality health care outcomes, then define them and pay to achieve them. There must be a culture of measurable performance improvement that permeates our country's health care system.

19. **Support the Patient-Centered Outcomes Research Institute (PCORI)**: This institute was created in the ACA, and consists of a Board of Governors and assisted by expert advisory panels that would analyze the best available scientific evidence and research, and make recommendations to the health care industry on what types of treatments are the most scientifically sound. This is not rationing of care, but the focusing on more rational care. This is the use of appropriate scientific evidence by both the physician and the patient at the point of care for informed and shared decision-making.

20. **Implement a Health Care Board**: This independent body of national experts would review health care costs and the best available scientific evidence, and make recommendations to the Centers of Medicare and Medicaid Services, all insurance companies, HHS, and Congress on what prices and procedures are reasonable for health care expenditures. This would be for all aspects of the health care system. This must be done so we can start to depoliticize the process of reasonable price setting based on value.

21. **Continue Major Insurance Reform**: Per the ACA, major insurance reform must continue. There must be a permanent stop to annual and lifetime caps on insurance expenditures, rescissions based on people getting serious medical problems, and denials for preexisting medical problems. There needs to be transparency in the health insurance industry to health care costs, profit, and medical loss ratios. We must stop paying for more and getting less. The ACA got this right and there must be relentless, ongoing reform to the insurance industry.

22. **Fix Medicare**: Medicare is a good public insurance plan for our elderly and disabled American citizens. However, it is bloated, inefficient, and has perverse payment. By realigning Medicare payments on value rather than on price/cost and by focusing on health generating outcomes and not just volume or procedures, appropriate cost control will be achieved. The price settings of the Medicare evaluation and management services and procedural costs are at the core of our cost crisis. If we gain control of appropriately repricing these services based on value then large cost reduction will be achieved. This becomes doubly important as private insurance company pricing uses Medicare pricing as a basis on which they arrive at their payment structure.

23. **Perform Administrative Simplification**: Our health care system is the most administratively complex in the world. There are papers and forms for everything. This extends to physicians, nurses, patients, billing, insurance, medications, medical devices, and everything in between. There must be electronic simplification so that all pertinent information can immediately download and populate all necessary data fields to simplify, streamline, and bring increased efficiency to a health care system that is drowning in paperwork.

24. **Legislate Liability Reform**: Our health care system is the most litigious system in the world, resulting in an excessive practice of "defensive medicine." The fear of making a mistake or not doing "enough" leads to more being done than is otherwise medically necessary. We must develop meaningful criteria for tort reform, caps on noneconomic damages, and alternative dispute resolution mechanisms. Caps on what lawyers get paid in handling these cases must also be established to stop exorbitant malpractice suits from being filed and large sums of money going to the lawyers and not the patients they are representing.

25. **Encourage Community-Based Care:** Moving more care into community-based clinics and home-based care must happen. We need to have less reliance on emergency rooms and hospitals as primary sources of care. They are default sources of care now because of the inadequate number of clinics that can provide primary care access points. ERs and hospitals will always be necessary for true emergencies and for patients that need hospitalization, but keeping people in their communities and homes healthy, and accessing more appropriate sources of care and not needing higher cost health care is our goal.

26. **Discuss End-of-Life Care**: Primary care physicians and other health care providers must be empowered to engage proactively with their patients, and the patient's families when appropriate, around end of life discussions. Preferences and options must be sensitively, compassionately, and realistically discussed so that the patient's preferences and desires are followed. This alignment of the patient's wishes will result in the right care being provided to the patient in the right place, at the right time, and for

the right reasons. This will result in markedly less health care system utilization and cost while honoring the person's desires.

27. **Maximize Input from the Women of America**: Women (mothers, wives, daughters of elderly parents) are critically important when forming an effective health care system. They collectively make more decisions concerning health care than doctors, nurses, or insurance companies. Working hand-in-hand with women to maximize their family's health and how to know when further help from their patient-centered medical home (PCMH) is needed will arm these important decision-makers with the basic skills to partner with their primary care providers and in turn the rest of the health care system.

28. **Investigate Innovative Pilots**: America must not be afraid to experiment and innovate around different health care models. This must be done through differing pilots to test effective models for health care delivery, quality, access, patient and practice satisfaction, health care outcomes, payment reform, and cost. Learning from these pilots and developing evidence-based best practices will go a long way towards propelling America into our new health care future. We need to continuously learn and grow as we evolve our future health care culture.

29. **Focus on Performance Improvement**: Our focus going forward should be vigilant performance improvement to dial in the outcomes we want to achieve. Our actions should be to refine and refocus, not to repeal and replace. This is the right path and we should have the courage and the boldness to stay on it.

30. Give it Time: America must be patient with this process. It took us 100 years to develop the health care system we have. It will take us at least 20 years of constant work to heal and "re-form" our fractured health care system from what America has to a much more flexible, accessible, affordable, quality health care system that we will need.

And now, there is one final signpost on the path I'd like to point out. This signpost is critically important as we continue the fight for a better health care system in America:

31. Restore Medicine as a Profession: A crucial step on the path forward involves restoring medicine as a profession instead of its current default state of being primarily a lucrative business. Physicians hold the critical key to dispelling much of the miasma of the U.S. health care system. Our nation's physicians must take the field in this critical battle and return medicine back to its birthright as a profession. Nobody else can do this for us. If we abrogate this responsibility and defer to the economists and politicians to guide us through the regulatory/implementation mist to the "better business" of health care, we will truly lose our last great opportunity to get this right. I remain optimistic that our nation's physicians have the collective will to see our noble calling of medicine shine as a profession and not exist merely as a business. We must refocus on our collective service to others if we are to restore people's hope, their dignity, and their health. This commitment from our nation's physicians is essential if we are to heal our fractured health care system.

Any one of the steps outlined above will move our health care system in the right direction. If all of these steps are followed, we will truly change health care in America in very positive and beneficial ways. If this path is followed, we will heal our fractured health care system. If it is not, we will continue along the path of our current expensive, underperforming, inefficient, disease care system and to the cliff at the end of the trail. The signposts are standing there before us, pointing to a more promising way. The choice is ours to make. Are we inevitably doomed to watch our health care system struggle and our citizens slide into decreasing health, or are we ready to treat our fractures, heal our wounds, and move forward to a healthier future? Do we have the collective will as a nation to make the changes needed? Time will tell.

Health care reform has been an exhaustive, all-out national battle over the last four years. It has been rancorous and downright mean-spirited, to say the least. I believe it has polarized us as a nation both in our political system and as fellow Americans. The anger, the fear, the hostility, the confusion, and the lies have served to convince me of the urgent need for health care reform. It is much needed, and long overdue. It is a fiscal imperative since the economic effect of health care is the most potent force threatening the solvency of our nation. As many Americans as possible must collectively embrace health care reform as a common good. By doing so we will become a fiscally safer, healthier, and more productive country, better able to compete with the rest of the world. We must keep our businesses strong by not having them overpay for health insurance, and we must keep our citizens healthy so that they can contribute to our workforce. We must provide safety and peace of mind to all by ensuring that people and their families do not go bankrupt over health care costs in a nation that is as plentiful and as full of promise as ours.

In the dark days of World War II, when England was on the brink of defeat and despair, Winston Churchill said, "Never, never, never give up!" So as a nation, we should never give up on what we believe is right for the health care of our citizens and for the good of our country. In many ways we are the best nation in the history of our world, and if we can now take health care to the next level, we will become even a better nation. It has been said that a nation's soul is in its people's keeping. Let our future generations speak proudly of what we as Americans collectively did to ensure a better health care system for those who would follow us. Let them be proud that at a moment of indecision and uncertainty we boldly moved forward with courage and conviction to heal our fractured health care system and to build a world-class health care system; one that not only propelled America's health forward, but also led to improved health for the world. Let us be proud that the soul and character of a country that was given to us for keeping was passed forward wisely and compassionately. For this we will be a better nation.

When health is absent,
wisdom cannot reveal itself,
art cannot manifest,
strength cannot fight,
wealth becomes useless,
and intelligence cannot be applied

– Herophilus, Ancient Greek Physician
335-280 BC

References

CHAPTER ONE

1. U.S. Census Bureau. Income, Poverty, and Health Insurance Coverage in the United States. September 16, 2010 [www.census.gov].

CHAPTER TWO

1. World Health Organization (WHO). [http://www.who.int/whr/2008/en/index.html].

2. The Commonwealth Fund Commission on a High Performance Health System, Why Not the Best? Results from the National Scorecard on U.S. Health System Performance, 2008. The Commonwealth Fund, July 2008 [http://www.commonwealthfund.org/publications/publications_show.htm?doc_id=692682].

3. McGinnis JM, Foege WH. Actual Causes of Death in the United States. *JAMA* 1993;270:2207-12.

4. Mokdad AH, Marks JS, Stroup DF, Gereberding JL. Actual Causes of Death in the United States, 2000. *JAMA* 2004;291:1230-1245.

5. White KL, Williams TF, Greenberg BG. The ecology of medical care. *N Engl J Med* 1961;265:885-892.

6. Green LA, Fryer GE, Yawn BP, Lanier D, Dovey SM. The ecology of medical care revisited. *N Engl J Med* 2001;344:2021-2025.

7. U.S. Census Bureau. Income, Poverty, and Health Insurance Coverage in the United States. September 16, 2010 [www.census.gov].

8.   Beal AC, Doty MM, Hernandez SE, Shea KK, Davis K. Closing the Divide: How Medical Homes Promote Equity in Health Care: Results From The Commonwealth Fund 2006 Health Care Quality Survey. The Commonwealth Fund, June 2007.

9.   Centers for Medicare & Medicaid Services. NHE Fact Sheet. [http://www.cms.hhs.gov/NationalHealthExpendData/25_NHE_Fact_Sheet.asp#TopOfPage]

10.   Centers for Medicare & Medicaid Services. NHE Fact Sheet. [http://www.cms.hhs.gov/NationalHealthExpendData/25_NHE_Fact_Sheet.asp#TopOfPage]

11.   The White House. Office of the Press Secretary. Remarks by the President at the Opening of the White House Forum on Health Reform. March 5, 2009. [http://www.whitehouse.gov/the_press_office/Remarks-by-the-President-at-the-Opening-of-the-White-House-Forum-on-Health-Reform].

12.   Himmelstein DU, Thorne D, Warren E, Woolhandler S. Medical Bankruptcy in the United States, 2007: Results of a National Study. *The American Journal of Medicine*, Elsevier, 2009.

13.   The White House. Office of the Press Secretary. Remarks by the President at the Opening of the White House Forum on Health Reform. March 5, 2009. [http://www.whitehouse.gov/the_press_office/Remarks-by-the-President-at-the-Opening-of-the-White-House-Forum-on-Health-Reform].

14.   Centers for Medicare and Medicaid Services. 2009 Annual Report of the Boards of Trustees of the Federal Hospital Insurance and Federal Supplementary Medical Insurance Trust Funds. Washington, DC, May 12, 2009 [http://www.cms.hhs.gov/ReportsTrustFunds/downloads/tr2009.pdf].

15.   U.S. Census Bureau News. U.S. Department of Commerce, Washington, DC. Facts for Features, Older Americans Month Celebrated in May. April 25, 2005. [http://www.census.gov/

Press-Release/www/releases/archives/facts_for_features_special_editions/004210.html]

16.   Medical Group Management Physician Compensation and Production Survey. 1998 and 2005.

17.   Association of American Medical Colleges. AAMC Reporter: December 2008. Graduates Report Higher Debt, Primary Care Interest. [http://www.aamc.org/newsroom/reporter/dec08/graduates.htm].

18.   Kaiser Family Foundation. Kaiser/HRET 2011 Employer Health Benefits Survey. September, 2011 [www.kff.org].

19.   Politico. Feder. September 28, 2011.

20.   WikiAnswers. What country in the world has most lawyers per capita? [http://wiki.answers.com/Q/What_country_in_the_world_has_most_lawyers_per_capita].

21.   Caroll. Going on the Offensive against Defensive Medicine. *Managed Care Magazine.* March 2005.

22.   McQuillan LJ, Abramyan H, Archi A. *Jackpot Justice: The True Cost of America's Tort System.* Pacific Research Institute, 2007.

23.   AMA Physicians Characteristics and Distribution 1980, 1990, 2000. Overpeck MD. Physicians in family practice 1931-67. *Public Health Rep* 1970; 85(6):485-494.

24.   Starfield B, Shi L, Macinko J. Contribution of Primary Care to Health Systems and Health. *The Millbank Quarterly,* 2005 Millbank Memorial Fund. Blackwell Publishing 2005; 83(3):457-502.

25.   World Health Organization (WHO). Responsiveness of Health Systems, Level and Distribution in all Member States, WHO Indexes, Estimates for 1999. The World Health Report 2000 [http://www.who.int/whr/2000/en/annex06_en.pdf].

26.   Medicare claims data; and Area Resource File, 2003.

27.   Gawande A. The Cost Conundrum: What a Texas town can

teach us about health care. *The New Yorker*. June 1, 2009.

CHAPTER THREE

1.   Covey, Stephen R. *The 8ᵗʰ Habit: From Effectiveness to Greatness*. FranklinCovey Co., 2004.

2.   Friedman, Thomas L. April 5, 2005. *The World is Flat: A Brief History of The Twenty-First Century*. United States: Farrar, Straus and Giroux.

3.   Fuchs, VR, Emanuel EJ. Health Care Reform: Why? What? When? *Health Affairs*, 24(6); 2005:1399-1414 [http://content. healthaffairs.org/cgi/content/full/24/6/1399].

4.   Bond, Michael T., Dobeck, Mark E., Knapp, Deborah Erdos. Using Health Savings Accounts to Provide Low-Cost Health Care. *Compensation Benefits Review* 2005 37: 29-32

5.   Health Affairs. The Health Insurance Picture in 1990 [http:// content.healthaffairs.org/cgi/reprint/10/2/104.pdf. The Kaiser Family Foundation. Employer Health Benefits 2009 Annual Survey. http://ehbs.kff.org/pdf/2009/7936.pdf].

6.   The White House. Office of the Press Secretary. Remarks by the President at the Opening of the White House Forum on Health Reform. March 5, 2009 [http://www.whitehouse.gov/the_press_of-fice/Remarks-by-the-President-at-the-Opening-of-the-White-House-Forum-on-Health-Reform].

7.   David U. Himmelstein, Elizabeth Warren, Deborah Thorne, and Steffie Woolhandler Himmelstein D. February 2, 2005. MarketWatch: Illness And Injury As Contributors To Bankruptcy. *Health Affairs* [http://content.healthaffairs.org/cgi/reprint/hlthaff. w5.63v1].

8.   U.S. Census Bureau. The 2010 Statistical Abstract. Table 102. Expectations of Life at Birth, 1970 to 2006, and Projections, 2010 to 2020 [http://www.census.gov/compendia/statab/2010/

tables/10s0102.pdf]. Centers for Disease Control and Prevention. Statistical Notes. Summary Measures of Population Health: Addressing the First Goal of Healthy People 2010, Improving Health Expectancy [http://www.cdc.gov/nchs/data/statnt/statnt21. pdf].

9.   U.S. Census Bureau, *Census 2000 Summary File 1 and 2010 Census Summary File 1.*

10.   Goldstein A, Damon B. We the American … Elderly. U.S. Department of Commerce Economics and Statistics Administration. Bureau of the Census. September 1993 [http://www.census.gov/apsd/wepeople/we-9.pdf].

Dartmouth Atlas [http://www.dartmouthatlas.org].

11.   Tanner M. The Grass is Not Always Greener, A Look at National Health Care Systems Around the World. CATO Institute Policy Analysis. March 18, 2008. No. 613:22-23

12.   World Health Organization (WHO). World Health Organization Assesses the World's Health Systems [http://www.who.int/whr/2000/media_centre/press_release/en/index.html].

13.   The Commonwealth Fund Commission on a High Performance Health System, Why Not the Best? Results from the National Scorecard on U.S. Health System Performance, 2008. The Commonwealth Fund, July 2008 [http://www.commonwealthfund.org/publications/publications_show.htm?doc_id=692682].

14.   Kaiser Family Foundation [http://www.kff.org/healthreform/upload/7914.pdf].

15.   Beal AC, Doty MM, Hernandez SE, Shea KK, Davis K. Closing the Divide: How Medical Homes Promote Equity in Health Care: Results From The Commonwealth Fund 2006 Health Care Quality Survey. The Commonwealth Fund, June 2007.

16.   Mead H, Cartwright-Smith L, Jones K, Ramos C, Siegel B, Woods K. Racial and Ethnic Disparities in U.S. Health Care: A

Chartbook. The Commonwealth Fund, March 13, 2008; 27.

17.   American Heart Association. Heart Disease and Stroke Statistics-2007 Update. Circulation, 2007; 1115:e69-e171.

18.   Wikipedia. The Pacific Railway Act of 1862 [http://en.wikipedia.org/wiki/Pacific_Railway_Acts].

19.   Chun-Ju Hsiao, Ph.D.; Paul C. Beatty, Ph.D.; Esther S. Hing, M.P.H.; David A. Woodwell, B.A.; Elizabeth A. Rechtsteiner, M.S.; and Jane E. Sisk, Ph.D., Division of Health Care Statistics. December 2009. Electronic Medical Record/Electronic Health Record Use by Office-based Physicians: United States, 2008 and Preliminary 2009 [http://www.cdc.gov/nchs/data/hestat/emr_ehr/emr_ehr.pdf]

20.   Centers for Disease Control. National Health Care Surveys. July 2008 [http://www.cdc.gov/nchs/data/infosheets/infosheet_nhcs.pdf].

21.   Centers for Disease Control. National Health Care Surveys. July 2008 [http://www.cdc.gov/nchs/data/infosheets/infosheet_nhcs.pdf].

22.   Institute of Medicine of the National Academies. Consensus Report. November 1, 1999. To Err is Human: Building A Safer Health System.

23.   The Commonwealth Fund Commission on a High Performance Health System. Why Not the Best? Results from a National Scorecard on U.S. Health System Performance. September 20, 2006, 34 [http://www.commonwealthfund.org/Content/Publications/Fund-Reports/2006/Sep/Why-Not-the-Best—Results-from-a-National-Scorecard-on-U-S—Health-System-Performance.aspx].

24.   PDFzone. Amicore boasts new electronic medical records system [http://www.pdfzone.com/c/a/Document-Management/Amicore-boasts-new-electronic-medical-records-system/].

25.   Steinbrook, Robert. Health Care Reform in Massachusetts: Expanding Coverage, Escalating Costs. *N Engl J Med* 2008 358: 2757-2760.

26.   Steinbrook, Robert. Health Care Reform in Massachusetts -- Expanding Coverage, Escalating Costs. *N Engl J Med* 2008 358: 2757-2760.

27.   Starfield B, Shi L, Macinko J. Contribution of Primary Care to Health Systems and Health. *The Millbank Quarterly,* 2005 Millbank Memorial Fund. Blackwell Publishing 2005; 83(3):457-502.

28.   American Medical Association. Health Care Trends 2008 [http://www.ama-assn.org/ama1/pub/upload/mm/409/2008-trends. pdf].

29.   American Academy of Family Physicians. National Resident Matching Program, 2010 Match Summary and Analysis [http://www.aafp.org/online/en/home/residents/match.html].

30.   Smart DR, Sellers J. Physician Characteristics and Distribution: 2008 Edition. Chicago, IL; American Medical Association; 2008.

31.   *JAMA.* 2000; 248(10): 1284-1289.

32.   Truman SR. Spokesman Review. September 13, 1949.

33.   Smith, WE. *LIFE.* Pages 115-126; September 20, 1948.

34.   Chairman Millis Js. The graduate education of physicians. Report of the Citizens Commission on Graduate Medical Education. Chicago: American Medical Association, 1966: 37.

35.   Rosenberg M. Columbia Nursing Dean Hopes to Transform Profession. Education Update Online, October 2002 [http://www. educationupdate.com/archives/2002/oct02/issue/med-columbia. htm].

36.   R. E. Mitchell : Evaluating The Clinical Preparation Of Physician Assistant Versus Nurse Practitioner Students And

The Characteristics Of Their Preceptors . The Internet Journal of Academic Physician Assistants. 2004 Volume 4 Number 1

CHAPTER FOUR

1.   Kaiser Family Foundation. Focus on Health Reform. National Health Insurance—A Brief History of Reform Efforts in the U.S. March 2009 [http://www.kff.org/healthreform/7871.cfm].

2.   Flexner A. Medical Education in the United States and Canada. A Report to the Carnegie Foundation for the Advancement of Teaching. 1910 [http://www.carnegiefoundation. org/publications/medical-education-united-states-and-canada-bulletin-number-four-flexner-report-0].

3.   Truman HS. 192 Special Message to the Congress Recommending a Comprehensive Health Program. November 19, 1945. Harry S. Truman Library & Museum [http://www.trumanli-brary.org/publicpapers/index.php?pid=483&st=&st1=].

4.   Daschle T, Greenberger S, Lambrew J. *Critical: What We Can Do About the Health Care Crisis.* 2008: 53

5.   Daschle T, Greenberger S, Lambrew J. *Critical: What We Can Do About the Health Care Crisis.* 2008: 53

6.   Daschle T, Greenberger S, Lambrew J. *Critical: What We Can Do About the Health Care Crisis.* 2008: 59

7.   Daschle T, Greenberger S, Lambrew J. *Critical: What We Can Do About the Health Care Crisis.* 2008: 62

8.   Daschle T, Greenberger S, Lambrew J. *Critical: What We Can Do About the Health Care Crisis.* 2008: 63

9.   Kennedy EM. The Cause of My Life. Inside the Fight for Universal Health Care. *Newsweek*, July 18, 2009 [http://www. newsweek.com/id/207406].

10.   Kaiser Family Foundation. Focus on Health Reform. *National*

Health Insurance—A Brief History of Reform Efforts in the U.S. March 2009: 6 [http://www.kff.org/healthreform/7871.cfm].

11.   Daschle T, Greenberger S, Lambrew J. *Critical: What We Can Do About the Health Care Crisis.* 2008:71

12.   Connolly C, Allen M. Medicare Drug Benefit May Cost $1.2 Trillion. Estimate Dwarfs Bush's Original Price Tag. *Washington Post*, February 9, 2005: A01 [http://www.washington-post.com/wp-dyn/articles/A9328-2005Feb8.html].

13.   AARP. Medicare Prescription Drug Coverage: Part I. November 10, 2009 [http://bulletin.aarp.org/yourhealth/medicare/articles/how_medicare_part_d_drug_coverage_works.html].

14.   Centers for Medicare and Medicaid Services. Medicare and You 2010. [http://www.medicare.gov/Publications/Pubs/pdf/10050.pdf].

15.   Veterans Affairs Health Care System [http://www1.va.gov/VETDATA/Pocket-Card/4X6_spring10_sharepoint.pdf].

16.   Military Health System [http://www.health.mil/About_MHS/Organizations/MHS_Offices_and_Programs/IIP/overview.asp].

17.   Indian Health System [http://info.ihs.gov/].

CHAPTER FIVE

1.   Reid, TR. *The Healing of America: A Global Quest for Better, Cheaper, and Fairer Health Care.* The Penguin Press, New York, 2009; P17-21.

2.   The Organization for Economic Co-operation and Development. Total Expenditure on Health Care as a Percentage of GDP. OECD Health Data 2007: Statistics and Indicators for 30 Countries. Paris: OECD, July 2007; 2004 Data.

3.   The Commonwealth Fund. *Average Spending on Health*

Per Capita. International Comparison of Spending on Health, 1980-2006 [http://www.commonwealthfund.org/ Content/Charts/ Report/The-Path-to-a-High-Performance-US-Health-System-A-2020-Vision-and-the-Policies-to-Pave-the-Way/International-Comparison-of-Spending-on-Health-1980-2006.aspx].

4.   Thompson, G. Health Expenditure: International Comparisons. Library House of Commons June 25, 2009;2:3

5.   The Commonwealth Fund. Percentage of National Health Expenditures Spent on Insurance Administration, *2005.* Commonwealth Fund Commission on a High Performance Health System, Why Not the Best? Results from the National Scorecard on U.S. Health System Performance, 2008. New York: The Commonwealth Fund, July 2008; 12, 34 [http://www.commonwealthfund.org/Content/Charts/Issue-Brief/How-Health-Care-Reform-Can-Lower-the-Costs-of-Insurance-Administration/Percentage-of-National-Health-Expenditures-Spent-on-Insurance-Administration-2005.aspx].

6.   2009 CMS Data Compendium. [http://www.cms.hhs.gov/ DataCompendium/15_2009_Data_Compendium.asp#TopOfPage].

7.   GAO report. [http://www.gao.gov/new.items/d05839r.pdf].

8.   2007 Health Care-Economist. [http:// healthcare-economist.com/2007/11/02/ private-health-insurance-and-administrative-expenses].

9.   2005 Milliman Report. [http://www.cahi.org/cahi_contents/resources/pdf/CAHIMedicareTechnicalPaper.pdf].

10.   Reid, TR. *The Healing of America: A Global Quest for Better, Cheaper, and Fairer Health Care.* The Penguin Press, New York, 2009; P37.

11.   The Commonwealth Fund. *Coronary Bypass Procedures per 100,000 Population, 2006.* [http://www. commonwealthfund.org/Content/Charts/Chartbook/ Multinational-Comparisons-of-Health-Systems-Data--2008/C/

Coronary-Bypass-Procedures--per-100-000-Population--2006.
aspx].

12.   The Organization for Co-operation and Development.
Number of MRI Units and CT Scanners per Million People.
OECD Health Data, 2007 Statistics and Indicates for 30 Countries.
Paris: OECD, July 2007.

13.   Reid, TR. *The Healing of America: A Global Quest for Better,
Cheaper, and Fairer Health Care.* The Penguin Press, New York, 2009;
P92.

14.   World Health Organization (WHO). Responsiveness
of Health Systems, Level and Distribution in all Member States,
WHO Indexes, Estimates for 1999. The World Health Report 2000
[http://www.who.int/whr/2000/en/annex06_en.pdf].

15.   World Health Organization (WHO). Fairness of Financial
Contribution to Health Systems in all Member States, WHO
Index, Estimates for 1997. The World Health Report 2000 [http://
www.who.int/whr/2000/en/annex07_en.pdf].

16.   The Commonwealth Fund. Life Expectancy at Birth, 2006.
[http://www.commonwealthfund.org/Content/Charts/Chartbook/
Multinational-Comparisons-of-Health-Systems-Data--2008/L/
Life-Expectancy-at-Birth--2006.aspx].

17.   Reid, TR. *The Healing of America: A Global Quest for Better,
Cheaper, and Fairer Health Care.* The Penguin Press, New York, 2009;
P32.

18.   Nolte et al., Ellen. "Measuring the Health of Nations:
Updating an Earlier Analysis," *Health Affairs*, January/February
2008, p71.

19.   The Commonwealth Fund. Multinational Comparisons of
Health Systems Data, November 2006.

20.   Schoen et al. "U.S. Health System Performance."

21.   K. Davis, C. Schoen, S.C. Schoenbaum, M.M. Doty, A.L.

Holmgren, J.L. Kriss, and K.K. Shea. Mirror, Mirror: Ranking of Six Nations. Mirror, Mirror on the Wall: An International Update on the Comparative Performance of American Health Care. The Commonwealth Fund, May 2007. [http://www.common-wealthfund.org/Content/Publications/Fund-Reports/2007/May/Mirror--Mirror-on-the-Wall--An-International-Update-on-the-Comparative-Performance-of-American-Healt.aspx].

22. Tanner M. The Grass is Not Always Greener, A Look at National Health Care Systems Around the World, March 18, 2008. CATO Institute Policy Analysis. No. 613:5

23. Tanner M. The Grass is Not Always Greener, A Look at National Health Care Systems Around the World, March 18, 2008. CATO Institute Policy Analysis. No. 613:8

24. The World Health Organization (WHO). Highlights on Health in France, 2004:30 [http://www.euro.who.int/document/E88547.pdf].

25. Tanner M. The Grass is Not Always Greener, A Look at National Health Care Systems Around the World, March 18, 2008. CATO Institute Policy Analysis. No. 613:13.

26. Tanner M. The Grass is Not Always Greener, A Look at National Health Care Systems Around the World, March 18, 2008. CATO Institute Policy Analysis. No. 613:14.

27. Reid, TR. *The Healing of America: A Global Quest for Better, Cheaper, and Fairer Health Care.* The Penguin Press, New York, 2009; P84.

28. Tanner M. The Grass is Not Always Greener, A Look at National Health Care Systems Around the World, March 18, 2008. CATO Institute Policy Analysis. No. 613:16.

29. National Public Radio. [http://www.npr.org/templates/story/story.php?storyId=110997469].

30. Tanner M. The Grass is Not Always Greener, A Look at

National Health Care Systems Around the World, March 18, 2008. CATO Institute Policy Analysis. No. 613:18

31.   Tanner M. The Grass is Not Always Greener, A Look at National Health Care Systems Around the World, March 18, 2008. CATO Institute Policy Analysis. No. 613:22-23.

32.   National Public Radio. [http://www.npr.org/templates/story/story.php?storyId=110997469].

33.   Tanner M. The Grass is Not Always Greener, A Look at National Health Care Systems Around the World, March 18, 2008. CATO Institute Policy Analysis. No. 613:24.

34.   National Public Radio. [http://www.npr.org/templates/story/story.php?storyId=110997469].

35.   Tanner M. The Grass is Not Always Greener, A Look at National Health Care Systems Around the World, March 18, 2008. CATO Institute Policy Analysis. No. 613:25, 27.

36.   The Organization for Economic Co-operation and Development. Out of Pocket Health Care Spending per Capita (2006). OECD Health Data 2008. June 2008.

37.   National Public Radio. [http://www.npr.org/templates/story/story.php?storyId=110997469].

38.   Tanner M. The Grass is Not Always Greener, A Look at National Health Care Systems Around the World, March 18, 2008. CATO Institute Policy Analysis. No. 613:29-30.

39.   National Public Radio. [http://www.npr.org/templates/story/story.php?storyId=110997469].

40.   Tanner M. The Grass is Not Always Greener, A Look at National Health Care Systems Around the World, March 18, 2008. CATO Institute Policy Analysis. No. 613:32-33.

41.   The Kaiser Family Foundation. Health Insurance Coverage for Total Population, states (2007-2008), U.S. (2008.) State Health Facts.org. [http://www.statehealthfacts.org/comparetable.

jsp?ind=125&cat=3].

42.   Reid, TR. *The Healing of America: A Global Quest for Better, Cheaper, and Fairer Health Care.* The Penguin Press, New York, 2009; 27.

43.   Tanner M. The Grass is Not Always Greener, A Look at National Health Care Systems Around the World, March 18, 2008. CATO Institute Policy Analysis. No. 613:34-35.

44.   Gawande, A. Testing, Testing. *The New Yorke*r, December 14, 2009.

CHAPTER SIX

1.   Kaiser Health Tracking Poll. Public Opinion on Health Care Issues. The Henry J. Kaiser Family Foundation. April 2010 [www.kff.org].

2.   Congressional Budget Office. Health Care [http://www.cbo.gov/publications/collections/health.cfm].

3.   Klein E. CBO: Health-care reform bill cuts deficit by $1.3 trillion over 20 years, covers 95 percent. The Washington Post, March 18, 2010 [http://voices.washingtonpost.com/ezra-klein/2010/03/cbo_health-care_reform_bill_cu.html].

4.   Franklin & Eleanor Roosevelt Institute. The Second Inaugural Address. January 20, 1937 [http://merchant.videotex.net/common/news/details.cfm?QID=2090&clientid=11005].

5.   Halvorson G. *Health Care Reform Now! A Prescription for Change.* Jossey-Bass Publications, San Francisco, California. August 2007.

CHAPTER SEVEN

1.   The White House. Office of the Press Secretary. Remarks by the President at the Opening of the White House Forum on Health

Reform. March 5, 2009. [http://www.whitehouse.gov/the_press_office/Remarks-by-the-President-at-the-Opening-of-the-White-House-Forum-on-Health-Reform].

2.   Madison J. Federalist No. 10. November 22, 1787.

3.   Hartman M, Martin A, et al. *Health Affairs* 2009;28:1;246-261

4.   American Hospital Association. Fast Facts on US Hospitals. November 11, 2009.

5.   World Health Organization (WHO). Top Ten Countries by Number of Physicians [http://www.who.int/whosis/database/core/core_select_process.cfm#].

6.   American Medical Association. AMA agenda for health system reform. February 2010.

7.   Centers for Disease Control and Prevention. FastStats. Nursing Home Care. 2004 National Nursing Home Survey: Facilities, table 1; Residents, table 13 [http://www.cdc.gov/nchs/fastats/nursingh.htm].

8.   U.S. Census Bureau. Newsroom—Older Americans Month Celebrated in May. April 19, 2002 [http://www.census.gov/Press-Release/www/releases/archives/facts_for_features_special_editions/000807.html]

9.   Bureau of Labor Statistics. Occupational Outlook Handbook, 2010-11 Edition [http://www.bls.gov/oco/ocos072.htm].

10.   Bureau of Labor Statistics. Registered Nurses. July 31, 2011. [www.bls.gov/oco/ocos083.htm]

11.   Medical Device and Diagnostic Industry (MD&DI) Magazine. 2009 MedTech Snapshot: Manufacturing: FDA Outreach Boosts the Number of U.S. Device Firms. December 2009 [http://www.mddionline.com/article/2009snapshot/manufacturing].

12.   Cornell University ILR School. Catherwood Library. Question of the Month. November 2, 2006 [http://www.ilr.cornell.

edu/library/research/questionOfTheMonth/nov06.html].

13.   U.S. Census Bureau. Statistics about Business Size (including Small Business) [http://www.census.gov/epcd/www/smallbus.html].

14.   Patient Centered Primary Care Collaborative (PCPCC) [http://www.pcpcc.net/files/PCPCCbrochure.pdf].

15.   Vital Information on Small Businesses [http://www.manta.com].

16.   Hatch OG, Blackwell JK, Klukowski KA. *The Wall Street Journal.* Why the Health Care Bills are Unconstitutional. January 2, 2010 [http://online.wsj.com/article/SB10001424052748703278604574624021919432770.html].

CHAPTER EIGHT

1.   Senate Finance Committee Chairman Max Baucus (D-Montana). Call to Action—Health Reform 2009. November 8, 2008.

2.   Arvantes J. President Obama Signs Legislation Expanding SCHIP Coverage to 4 Million More Children. AAFP News Now. February 6, 2009.

3.   Herszenhorn DM, Hulse C. Deal Reached in Congress on $789 Billion Stimulus Plan. *The New York Times.* February 12, 2009.

4.   The White House, Office of the Press Secretary. White House Forum on Health Reform. Washington, DC. March 5, 2009.

5.   YouTube. White House Summit Statement. March 5, 2009 [http://www.youtube.com/watch?v=3DTT6EmhmN0&feature=PlayList&p=5EF785D79069501F&index=15].

6.   The Henry Kaiser Family Foundation. Focus on Health Reform—Side by Side Comparison of Major Health Care, Reform Proposals. December 23, 2009.

7.   The Commonwealth Fund. Starting on the Path to a High

Performance Health System: Analysis of Health System Reform Provisions of Reform Bills in the House of Representatives and Senate. December 2009.

8.   Washington Post.com. Health Care Reform: How the Bills Stack Up. December 20, 2009.

9.   Associated Press. 50 million new patients? Expect doc shortages. *Revamped health care system could swamp primary care physicians.* MSNBC; September 13, 2009 [http://www.msnbc.msn.com/id/32829974/ns/health-health_care/].

10.   National Association of Community Health Centers. May 2010 [http://www.nachc.org].

11.   White House. HR 3288—Consolidated Appropriations Act, 2010 [http://www.whitehouse.gov/the-press-office/pending-legislation/HR-3288].

12.   The Congressional Budget Office. The Long-Term Outlook for Health Care Spending. November 2007 [http://www.cbo.gov/ftpdocs/87xx/doc8758/MainText.3.1.shtml].

13.   The White House, Office of Public Engagement. Protecting Consumers Through Health Insurance Reform. December 17, 2009.

14.   McQuillan LF, Abramyan H, Archie A. *Jackpot Justice: The True Cost of America's Tort System.* Pacific Research Institute, 2007.

CHAPTER NINE

1.   Tumulty K. Mass Mutiny. Scott Brown's surprise Senate win in the Bay State may have derailed Obama's health care reform. *Time* magazine, February 1, 2010: 30-31.

2.   The White House. Remarks by the President in State of the Union Address. Office of the Press Secretary, January 27, 2010 [http://www.whitehouse.gov/the-press-office/remarks-president-state-union-address].

3.   The White House. Health Care. The President's Proposal for Health Reform. March 21, 2010 [http://www.whitehouse.gov/issues/health-care].

4.   The White House. Remarks by the President and Vice President at Signing of the Health Insurance Reform Bill. Office of the Press Secretary, March 23, 2010 [http://www.whitehouse.gov/the-press-office/remarks-president-and-vice-president-signing-health-insurance-reform-bill].

5.   The Henry J. Kaiser Family Foundation. Summary of New Health Reform Law. Publication #8061, March 26, 2010 [www.KPF.org].

6.   Klein, E. CBO: Health Care Reform Bill Cuts Deficit by $1.3 Trillion Over 20 Years, Covers 95 percent. Washington Post, March 18, 2010 [http://voices.washingtonpost.com/ezra-klein/2010/03/cbohealth-carereformbillcu.html].

CHAPTER TEN

1.   Beal AC, Doty MM, Hernandez SE, Shea KK, Davis K. Closing the Divide: How Medical Homes Promote Equity in Health Care: Results From The Commonwealth Fund 2006 Health Care Quality Survey. The Commonwealth Fund, June 2007.

2.   Gawande A. Testing, Testing. *The New Yorker*, December 14, 2009.

3.   Institute of Medicine. To Err is Human. Building a Safer Health System. National Academy of Sciences. November 1999.

4.   Luther King M., Jr. Presentation at the Second National Convention of the Medical Committee for Human Rights. Chicago, March 25, 1966.

5.   Medicare claims data; and Area Resource File, 2003.

6.   The Patient Centered Medical Home. American Academy of Family Physicians. April 2009 [http://www.aafp.org].

7.   Council on Graduate Medical Education. 20th Report; General Recommendations. Minutes of Meeting, November 18 and 19, 2009 [http://www.cogme.gov/1109minutes.htm].

8.   Steiner BD et al. Community Care of North Carolina: Improving care through community health networks. Ann Fam Med 2008;6:361-367.

9.   Mercer. Executive Summary, 2008 Community Care of North Carolina Evaluation [http://www.communitycarenc. com/PDFDocs/Mercer percent20ABD percent20Report percent20SFY08.pdf].

10.   Institute for Healthcare Improvement. Health Partners uses "BestCare" practices to improve care and outcomes, reduce costs [http://www.ihi.org/NR/ rdonlyres/7150DBEF-3853-4390-BBAF-30ACDCA648F5/0/ IHITripleAimHealthPartnersSummaryofSuccessJul09.pdf].

11.   Geisinger Health System. Presentation at White House roundtable on Advanced Models of Primary Care. August 10, 2009.

12.   Institute for Healthcare Improvement. Genesys HealthWorks integrates primary care with health navigator to improve health, reduce costs [http://www.ihi.org/NR/ rdonlyres/2A19EFDB-FB9D-4882-9E23-D4845DC541D8/0/ IHITripleAimGenesysHealthSystemSummaryofSuccessJul09.pdf].

13.   Colorado Department of Health Care Policy and Financing. Colorado Medical Home [http://www.colorado.gov/cs/ Satellite?blobcol=urldata&blobheader=application percent2Fpdf&bl obkey=id&blobtable=MungoBlobs&blobwhere=1239162002481&s sbinary=true].

14.   Dorr DA, Wilcox AB, Brunker CP, et al. The effect of technology-supported, multidisease care management on the mortality and hospitalization of seniors. Findings updated for presentation at White House roundtable on Advanced Models of Primary Care. *J Am Geriatr Soc.* 2008;56(12):2195-202. August 10, 2009.

15.   Baron RJ, MD. What's Keeping Us So Busy in Primary Care? A Snapshot from One Practice. *New England Journal of Medicine*, April 29, 2010. Volume 362:1632, Number 17 [http://content.nejm.org/cgi/content/full/362/17/1632].

16.   *Health Affairs*. What Does It Cost Physician Practices To Interact With Health Insurance. May 14, 2009 [http://content.healthaffairs.org/cgi/content/abstract/hlthaff/28.4.w533].

17.   Halvorson G. Healthcare *Reform Now! A Prescription for Change*. Josey Bass. San Francisco, CA. 2007; 262-264

18.   Pollan M. *The Omnivore's Dilemma: A Natural History of Four Meals*. The Penguin Press, 2006 [http://www.michaelpollan.com/omnivore.php].

19.   Robert Graham Center. Workforce Data for AHRQ. Data in current publication [https://www.aamc.org/download/122862/data/phillips.pdf.pdf].

20.   The Commonwealth Fund. Average Spending on Health Per Capita. International Comparison of Spending on Health. 1980-2006 [http://www.commonwealthfund.org/Content/Charts/Report/The-Path-to-a-High-Performance-US-Health-System-A-2020-Vision-and-the-Policies-to-Pave-the-Way/International-Comparison-of-Spending-on-Health-1980-2006.aspx].

21.   World Health Organization (WHO). Responsiveness of Health Systems, Level and Distribution in all Member States, WHO Indexes, Estimates for 1999. The World Health Report 2000 [http://www.who.int/whr/2000/en/annex06_en.pdf].

22.   The Commonwealth Fund Commission on a High Performance Health System. Why Not the Best? Results from the National Scorecard on U.S. Health System Performance, 2008. The Commonwealth Fund, July 2008.

23.   Reid TR. *The Healing of America: A Global Quest for Better, Cheaper, and Fairer Health Care*. The Penguin Press, New York, 2009; P92.

24.   Tillinghast-Towers Perrin. U.S. Tort Costs: 2003 Update, Trends and Findings on the Cost of U.S. Tort System. 17(2003).

25.   Ibid.

26.   Brooke J. Doran, ed. Jury Verdict Research: Verdicts, Settlements and Statistical Analysis 5, 8. 2005.

27.   Mello M, Chandra A, Gawande A, Studdert D. National Costs of the Medical Liability System. *Health Affairs*, September 2010 (29):1569-1577.

28.   Sorrel AL. Physicians seek gains in state liability reforms; Additional Information: More doctors practice defensively, polls say. American Medical News, March 15, 2010 [http://www.ama-assn.org/amednews/2010/03/15/prl20315.htm].

29.   Caroll. Going on the Offensive against Defensive Medicine. *Managed Care Magazine*. March 2005.

30.   McQuillan LJ, Abramyan H, Archi A. *Jackpot Justice: The True Cost of America's Tort System*. Pacific Research Institute, 2007.

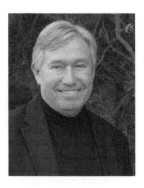

TED EPPERLY, MD, is a family physician in Boise, Idaho, where he sees patients, teaching family medicine residents, and directs the Family Medicine Residency of Idaho. He is a clinical professor of family and community medicine at the University of Washington School of Medicine and is a past president and chairman of the board of the American Academy of Family Physicians, which represents over 103,000 family physicians nationally. Dr. Epperly is the co-chair of the Center on Accountable Care of the Patient-Centered Primary Care Collaboration (PCPCC), which is comprised of over 1,000 organizations dedicated to transforming the United States health care system around primary care. He has also published over 50 articles and has given over 850 lectures and media interviews nationally and internationally on medical topics and health care reform and its importance.

For more information, please visit us at:
www.fracturedhealthcare.com

Photo taken by Michelle Robin

17358000R00192

Made in the USA
San Bernardino, CA
09 December 2014